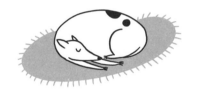

sleep

Relax, replenish and
rejuvenate with a new
approach to sleep

lisa varadi

Illustrations by Elda Broglio

Hardie Grant

QUADRILLE

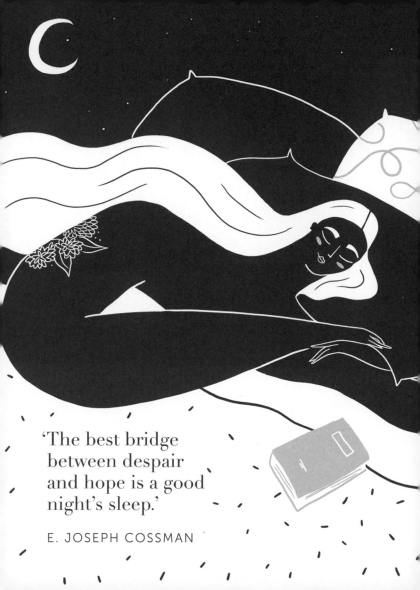

'The best bridge
between despair
and hope is a good
night's sleep.'

E. JOSEPH COSSMAN

CONTENTS

INTRODUCTION

Sleep is one of nature's greatest gifts. It is a time for our bodies to relax, replenish and rejuvenate. Sleep is essential to life, yet its value often goes unrecognized. Much like nutrition and exercise, sleep is vital to our functioning. It provides us with the energy we need to go about our day and enhances our ability to discover, experience and enjoy all that life has to offer.

While we sleep, our bodies are often still. It appears as if we are idle and void of all activity. In reality, there is quite a lot that is taking place; our minds are active and we may be immersed in a wonderful dream. Our bodies are mending from the stresses and exertions of the day. We are busy getting ready to relish in the joys and take on the challenges of what lies ahead.

Sleep is fundamental to our existence and we need to ensure that we are getting the right amount to keep us healthy and performing at our peak. Sadly, the pressures of modern times have made a good night's sleep very difficult to come by. Stress and worry keep many of us wide awake well into the night. In addition, the demands of everyday life often push sleep to the bottom of our list of priorities. For some, sleep has become a nuisance, a chore that must be completed.

The goal of this book is to raise awareness of both the significance and splendour of sleep. Upon reading it, you will gain a greater understanding of what sleep is, why we need it and how to obtain more of it. The tips and exercises I have provided are those that I have employed in my practice for a number of years.

Sleep is a splendid and tranquil state that should come to us effortlessly. Nature has awarded us this time to take a break, to process and to heal. The arrival of bedtime should be welcomed, not feared. Understanding what is typical and viewing sleep in a positive manner will help us to overcome any obstacles that we may encounter. Opening our minds and appreciating all of the benefits that come with deep and uninterrupted sleep will make us fall asleep more quickly once we have climbed into our beds.

Breathing, laughing, walking and taking delight in all of life's offerings will help us attain the sleep that our bodies need. When we live right, we will sleep tight!

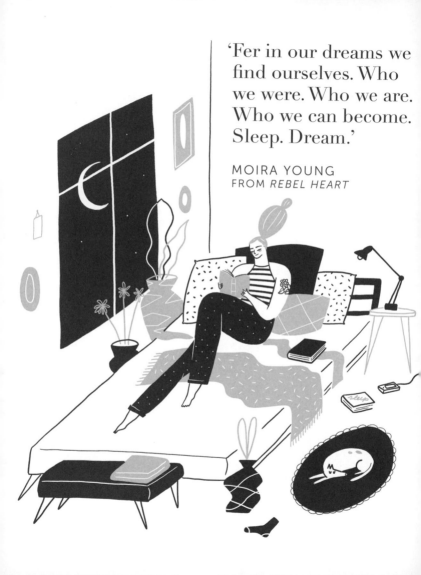

'Fer in our dreams we find ourselves. Who we were. Who we are. Who we can become. Sleep. Dream.'

MOIRA YOUNG
FROM *REBEL HEART*

THE STORY OF SLEEP

Sleep has been a source of fascination and wonderment for thousands of years. Throughout our history, physicians, philosophers and spiritual healers have all sought to explain how we sleep, as well as understand why we sleep. Their collective contributions paved the way for what we now know to be true: sleep is an active process that is essential to life.

The story of sleep begins with early humans. Our hunter-gatherer ancestors relied heavily on their internal body rhythms and external cues, such as the rising and setting of the sun, to determine when and how they slept. The sleep schedules of our early ancestors were also influenced by the weather, the search for food and the presence of danger. In the early years of human history, sleep usually took place on the ground within caves. Our ancestors would rely on foliage or other soft materials for comfort.

Despite our understanding of the sleep patterns of early humans, we know very little about their beliefs about sleep. Thousands of years would pass before there was any evidence of human sleep exploration. The ancient Egyptians were one of the earliest civilizations with documented views on sleep. Through hieroglyphics, we know that they valued sleep, and believed that the soul was able to travel beyond the physical body during sleep. Sleep was viewed as a means of communication with the Gods and the dead. Sleep was also a source of fear, as demons were able to frighten the living while they slept.

The people of ancient Egypt were one of the first to sleep on raised beds. Their beds were made of wood and the mattresses contained wool or straw. The legs of the beds were often carved to resemble those of animals, such as the paws of a lion. The headrests often displayed carvings of the Gods.

The ancient Greeks continued to believe that sleep served a divine purpose. However, during this time, academics were beginning to examine sleep in secular terms. The Greek philosopher Aristotle sought to understand sleep as a science. He stated that sleep is part of the digestive process. He also observed that sleep is not limited to humans but exhibited by much of the animal kingdom.

The ancient Romans viewed sleep in naturalistic terms. They valued early awakenings and continuous daytime activity was commended. Overall, sleep was viewed negatively, and physicians would advise against sleeping too much. The Romans did, however, view their bedrooms as places of tranquility and as sanctuaries from the stresses of everyday life.

In ancient India, sleep was believed to provide spiritual enlightenment and physical revitalization. The connection between sleep and health was described by Charaka, a prominent physician. He believed that both insufficient and excessive sleep are bad for health and longevity. He also stated that poor sleep and an unhealthy diet can lead to the development of disease.

The people of ancient India also placed great value on the direction in which a person slept. Sleeping with the head pointed north was the worst position and could result in sleep deprivation and illness. Sleeping with the head pointed south was the best position and would bring about refreshing sleep, happiness and longevity.

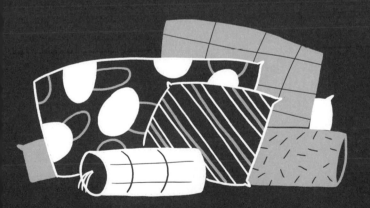

Sleep was considered to be of great value in ancient China. Many early Chinese thinkers described sleep as a time of communication with the soul. In addition, conditions arising from sleep difficulties were well described, including those that we recognize today as insomnia and sleep apnoea.

The allure of sleep continued into the Middle Ages and the Renaissance period. Sleep was a very prominent subject in the writings and paintings of the period. Some would portray the resemblance of sleep to death while others would emphasize the healing and calming powers of sleep. Among academics, there was increasing acceptance that the brain is the centre of sensation and consciousness.

All through human existence, there have been significant changes in sleep schedules and sleep patterns. The invention of the lightbulb saw a dramatic change in the timing of sleep. People were able to do far more after sunset than in previous centuries, and this resulted in later bedtimes.

Throughout history, many civilizations followed a sleep pattern quite unlike our own. Instead of one continuous sleep, people slept for approximately 4 hours, woke to carry out some light activity for an hour or two, and then slept for another 4 hours until daylight. This sleep schedule lasted until the Industrial Revolution of the 18th and 19th centuries, when a continuous 6- to 8-hour slumber was more conducive to the demands of society.

Ancient civilizations and the early modern era brought with them a number of important developments in the subject of sleep. However, many prominent thinkers believed sleep to be a passive process and that our bodies simply 'turn off' at night. During the late 19th century, the idea that sleep was a state of complete inactivity came to be questioned.

The last century has brought about significant advances in our knowledge of the processes that underlie sleep. Nathaniel Kleitman, a prominent sleep researcher in the mid-20th century, greatly progressed our understanding of the biological clock and the regulation of sleep. The last century also saw the identification and classification of a number of sleep disorders and the development of the electroencephalogram (EEG) to aid in their diagnosis. There have also been great advances in the treatment of many sleep disorders.

Although we have come a long way in our understanding of sleep, there is still much that is awaiting discovery. The field of sleep medicine is expanding at a rapid rate as new breakthroughs continue to be made. The beauty and mysticism surrounding sleep is still celebrated today in many cultures throughout the world. The subject will continue to captivate for years to come as the story of sleep is far from its conclusion.

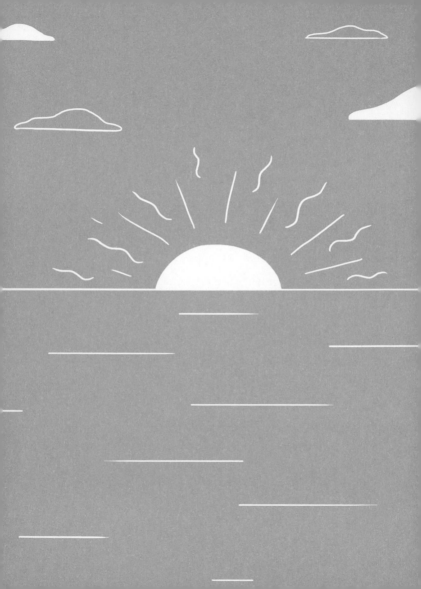

LET'S TALK ABOUT
THE BODY CLOCK

Our world is full of rhythms. The rising and setting of the sun, the waxing and waning of the tides and the changing of the seasons are examples of rhythms, or cycles, within our environment. They follow a sequence that we can observe and predict.

Not only are cycles present in our external world, but much of our internal physiology follows a rhythmic pattern. In fact, the brain houses a master rhythm, known as the circadian rhythm or circadian clock, that governs the inner processes that follow a daily cycle. Not surprisingly, sleep happens to be one of these processes.

Together, sleep and wakefulness combine to form what is known as the sleep-wake cycle. This is the 24-hour period within which we typically spend one-third of the time asleep and two-thirds of the time awake. Due to genetics, there may be some slight variation in the length of a person's circadian rhythm, but the average length is approximately 24 hours.

The circadian rhythm is regulated in a part of the brain called the suprachiasmatic nucleus (SCN). The SCN detects signals from the eyes regarding the amount of light or darkness. The SCN processes this information and then sends a signal to a gland at the base of the brain called the pineal gland. This gland secretes the sleep hormone melatonin in the presence of darkness. An increase in the secretion of melatonin at night tells the body that it's time to sleep.

The circadian rhythm is not fully established until the third or fourth month of life. This is why newborns wake frequently. When a child enters puberty, the circadian rhythm tends to shift slightly. This lasts for a few years and is one of the reasons why teenagers are more prone to having later bedtimes and being late risers.

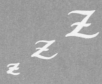

HOW TO BUMP THE EARLY
AFTERNOON SLUMP

We've all experienced the afternoon sleepiness that often follows lunchtime. Many of us are quick to blame the composition of the meal or our digestive tracts that are using all of the body's energy to break down food rather than maintain mental clarity.

Although eating a carbohydrate-rich meal can make matters worse, the food itself is not the underlying problem. The circadian clock has a natural 'dip' about 6 or 7 hours after we wake in the morning. Therefore, it is natural to feel tired around this time.

What can be done to offset this slump? Stepping outside for some fresh air and natural light or going for a short walk will help you regain your energy and focus. It's important to bear in mind that this tiredness usually doesn't last too long so your alertness and ability to concentrate will soon return.

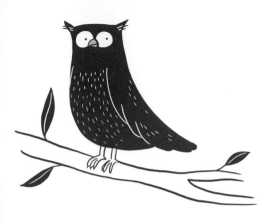

OWLS AND LARKS

In the land of the circadian clock there reside two types of people, the owls and the larks. Most of us fall within one of these two categories but some lie in between. The owls are those who are late to bed and late to rise. The larks are those who awaken early in the morning and tire early in the evening. The terms owl and lark are used to describe what is known as your chronotype.

Owls tend to struggle with the typical 9am–5pm work schedule. Waking up in the morning can be fairly challenging as can staying awake during the after-lunch slump. These difficulties often lead to a reliance on alarm clocks and caffeine to keep up with the weekday schedule. Owls tend to function at their best later in the day.

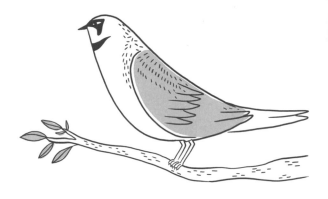

In contrast, larks are able to work harder and more efficiently in the mornings. They may begin to tire towards the end of the workday. Night shifts are a challenge for the lark and socializing and performing hobbies in the evenings are near-impossible pursuits. Larks will often push themselves well into the evening to keep up with the demands of the day.

A person's chronotype is largely determined by genetics, however lifestyle factors can have an influence. Habits, such as staying up too late, which you have followed over a long period, can impact the timing of your circadian rhythm. The key to survival is a sustainable balance between your daily schedule and your genetic make-up.

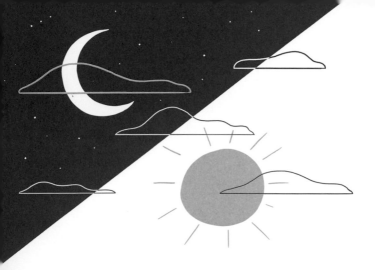

KEEPING UP THE BEAT

Since the circadian rhythm is so vital to our existence, it is essential that it is kept on track. This is the role of what are known as zeitgebers, external cues that help to harmonize our internal clock.

There are several environmental factors that help keep the body's master clock synchronized:

DAYLIGHT

Light is the primary zeitgeber because it is the most powerful regulator of the circadian rhythm. In the presence of daylight, melatonin production decreases and we become awake and alert. When daylight is absent, melatonin is secreted, and we become sleepy.

AMBIENT TEMPERATURE

A room that is uncomfortable (either too hot or too cold) can shift the circadian rhythm forward and delay the onset of sleep. Frequent waking and less time spent in deep sleep can also occur if the temperature of your sleep environment is not right.

EATING

The times at which we eat can help set our internal clock. Eating smaller meals throughout the day and avoiding heavy or spicy foods before bed can help to make sleep arrive at a proper time. Hunger hormones have a strong influence on the timing of the circadian rhythm. Trying to sleep with an empty stomach can delay sleep onset. Consuming a small nutritious snack before bedtime can offset the wakefulness-promoting effect of hunger.

PHYSICAL ACTIVITY

The timing of physical activity can help to set the circadian rhythm. Exercising at night can increase your body temperature and the secretion of the alertness-enhancing hormone adrenalin, both of which can make falling asleep very challenging. Exercising during the day, on the other hand, can improve your ability to fall asleep and stay asleep at night. Exercise has also been found to reduce the likelihood of developing certain sleep disorders, including insomnia, restless legs syndrome (RLS) and sleep apnoea.

WITH GREAT CAPABILITY COMES GREAT RESPONSIBILITY

The circadian clock is often referred to as the master clock, and for good reason. It has the immense task of regulating several cycles in addition to that of sleep and wakefulness.

BODY TEMPERATURE

Our core body temperature fluctuates throughout the day, reaching its peak in the late afternoon and its lowest point during the night, about 2 hours before we wake up. The steep decline in body temperature that occurs at night is essential for sleep to occur. The ideal time to go to bed is shortly after the start of this drop because following this 'sleep window', wakefulness increases, and it becomes more difficult to fall asleep. While we sleep, our body temperature drops even further. This helps us remain asleep and enter deep sleep.

HORMONE PRODUCTION AND SECRETION

Our hormone levels vary throughout the day. The amount of sleep hormone melatonin is at its highest during the night and its lowest level during daylight hours. The production and secretion of hormones that regulate mood, stress, appetite, metabolism and reproduction are heavily regulated by the circadian rhythm. Any disruption of the sleep-wake cycle can affect the secretion of these hormones and any disturbance in hormone secretion can alter the sleep-wake cycle.

IMMUNITY

The immune system is a highly intricate network designed to protect us from dangerous invaders. The formation and release of the immune cells that carry out this vital function fluctuate throughout the day. The levels of proinflammatory cytokines (such as Interleukin-1β (IL-1β), Interleukin-12 (IL-12) and Tumor Necrosis Factor-α (TNF-α) are higher at night, while the levels of anti-inflammatory cytokines (such as Interleukin-10 (IL-10)) and infection-fighting white blood cells are higher during the daytime.

HEART FUNCTION

The heart is vital to human life. It pumps blood that provides nourishment to our organs and tissues. In order to do its job properly, the heart must both contract and relax. Special cells of the heart, known as pacemaker cells, set the rhythm of the heart and tell it when it's time to contract. These pacemaker cells are directly controlled by the circadian clock. This means that sleep can influence heart function.

A CLOCK OF THEIR OWN

The synchrony of the human body is the key to our physiology. Not surprisingly it has been discovered that many organs and tissues have their own 'peripheral clocks'. These are localized clocks that regulate the frequency and duration of the activity of the organ or tissue. These clocks run fairly independently, but they do communicate with the SCN (see page 16) and the master clock does exert a bit of control.

LOCATIONS OF PERIPHERAL CLOCKS

- Lungs
- Liver
- Skin
- Fat cells
- Immune cells
- Kidneys
- Stomach
- Intestines
- Pancreas

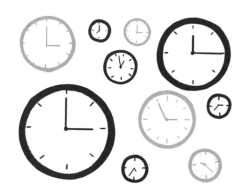

INCREASED MELATONIN +

INCREASED SLEEP PRESSURE = SLEEP

TO SLEEP OR NOT TO SLEEP?

The regulation of sleep is complex. The determination of when to sleep and when to wake is not carried out by the circadian rhythm alone. There is another key participant in the decision-making process. A system known as sleep-wake homeostasis helps to balance sleep and wakefulness. When a person has been awake for a long time, a drive for sleep (or sleep pressure) builds up, which tells the body that it's time to sleep. Sleep-wake homeostasis ensures that the longer you are awake and the more energy you expend, the sleepier you will be when bedtime approaches.

'Sleep that knits up the ravell'd sleeve of care,

The death of each day's life, sore labour's bath,

Balm of hurt minds, great nature's second course,

Chief nourisher in life's feast.'

WILLIAM SHAKESPEARE,
MACBETH ACT II,
SCENE II

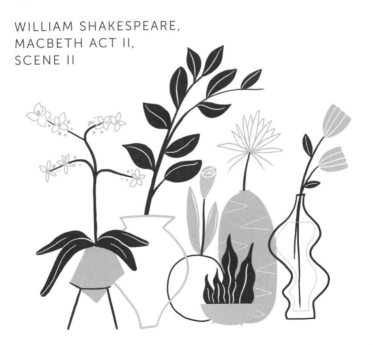

FROM SHALLOW TO DEEP, THERE ARE FOUR STAGES OF SLEEP

Once thought of as a time of complete inactivity, we now know sleep to be a dynamic process that progresses through different stages. These stages are marked by differences in brain activity and depth. An EEG measures the electrical activity in the brain and displays a picture in the form of waves. There are four stages of sleep.

STAGE 1

When we first drift off we enter stage 1. Here, we experience a light and more 'alert' type of sleep. This stage is often considered a state of transition between wakefulness and sleep. The body is in an extremely relaxed state. The brain waves that are seen at the very beginning of this stage are known as alpha waves and are slow and wide. As we drift further into sleep the brain waves change into what are known as theta waves. These waves have an even slower frequency than alpha waves. At the end of stage 1 the body is still in a period of very light sleep.

STAGE 2

This is similar to stage 1, in that the body is in a state of
light sleep and the person can be very easily roused.
However, during this stage, the body produces more rapid
and rhythmic brain waves known as sleep spindles. These
sleep spindles occur about every minute or two during
stage 2 of sleep. Another kind of wave that occurs during
this stage is called a k-complex. These often occur just
prior to, or shortly after, sleep spindles.

STAGE 3

This is when very slow waves, known as delta waves,
start to emerge. This stage is sometimes referred to as
delta sleep. At this point we are in deep sleep and are less
responsive to noises and activity in our environment. It is
also during this stage that the body enters its 'repair' mode.
Sleepwalking or bed-wetting tend to occur most often
during this sleep stage.

STAGE 4

Known as rapid eye movement (REM) sleep. The sleep stages described above are often collectively referred to as non-REM (NREM) sleep. REM derives its name from the fast movement of the eyes that occurs during this stage, as seen on a device known as an electrooculogram (EOG). Adults spend 20 per cent of their sleep time in REM sleep, while for infants it is up to 50 per cent. During REM sleep, brain activity is heightened while the voluntary muscles are immobilized. REM sleep is when most dreaming occurs.

Sleep does not progress through all the stages in order. When a person falls asleep they enter stage 1. They then go through stages 2 and 3, then back through stage 2, which is followed by REM sleep. Once REM is complete the sleeper enters stage 2 and the cycle repeats itself. You will usually go through five of these cycles per night, with the length of REM sleep increasing with each cycle. Once we fall asleep, it takes about 90 minutes for the body to go from stage 1 to REM sleep.

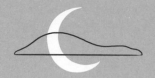

WHAT HAPPENS TO THE BODY
DURING THE SLEEP STAGES?

STAGE 1
Light sleep
Easily roused

STAGE 2
Body temperature drops
Heart rate slows
Breathing rate drops
Body is preparing to
  enter deep sleep

STAGE 3
Deep sleep
Difficult to rouse
Muscles are relaxed
Growth and repair
  of tissues

STAGE 4
Rapid eye movement
Heart rate quickens
Blood pressure rises
Breathing rate increases
Muscles are immobilized
Brain is more active
Most dreaming occurs

RIDING THE ALPHA WAVES

Alpha waves are those that occur when we are relaxed and resting with our eyes closed. They are seen very early on in stage 1 of sleep.

As it turns out, enhancing alpha wave activity has some health benefits. An increase in focus, attention and memory when learning new information or performing a task can be seen in those who show greater amounts of alpha brain wave activity. A decrease in symptoms of depression and anxiety have also been observed.

So how can we go about increasing our alpha waves? The best way to do so is to enter a mental state, or perform an exercise, which produces calmness. This will not only enhance the desired brain waves but also improve physical health and vitality.

MINDFULNESS

Mindfulness involves bringing your attention to the present moment. Focusing on your current surroundings and taking in all experiences in a nonjudgmental way allows for the release of tension and worry. In addition to enhancing alpha brain wave activity, practising mindfulness has been shown to reduce pain, anxiety and depression. Enhanced immune system function and improvements in focus, attention, sleep and feelings of overall wellbeing have also been observed in those who regularly engage in the practice.

MEDITATION

Meditation is a technique that is used to bring about a state of calmness, relaxation and mental clarity. It is usually performed seated or lying down. There are many types of meditation and several exercises can be performed. There are those that encourage focus and drawing one's attention to their own body, the present (mindfulness), an object or a tranquil place. Some involve visualizations, while others require emptying the mind of all thoughts. Those who meditate regularly experience enhanced mood, sleep and energy levels.

BREATHING

We all breathe to live, but most of us do not take the time to notice our breath. Breathing deeply and fully can elevate us to a higher level of consciousness, as well as to a deeper and more nourishing state of unconsciousness (sleep). Focused breathing can reduce stress and improve the health of the mind and body.

MOVEMENT

Our bodies are made to move. We use motion every day to complete tasks and to maintain our physical health. What many people don't know is that movement is also important for our emotional and spiritual wellbeing. Light motion can ease tension and calm the mind. Whether it's the smooth movements of our muscles as we stretch or the gentle glide of our hand as we softly stroke the fur of a pet, delicately moving about relaxes us and enables us to absorb all that surrounds us.

In the realm of sleep, we do not attain alpha status by way of assertion. We do so through mindfulness, acceptance and letting our tensions go.

ENHANCING YOUR INNER ALPHA

There are a number of exercises you can perform to help you reach the alpha zone.

EXERCISE 1: WATCHING THE WAVES

This is a simple visualization meditation exercise that will help get you into the alpha zone. You can do it wherever or whenever you like. When you are comfortable and ready, follow these steps:

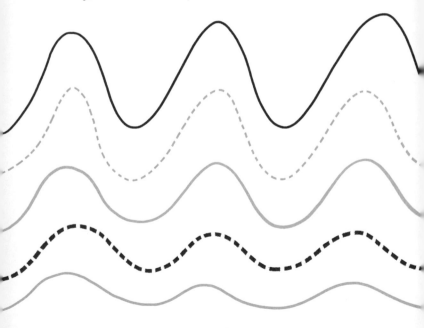

1. Close your eyes and place both of your hands on your abdomen.

2. Breathe in slowly and deeply, hold for 5 seconds, and then slowly exhale. Do three more of these breaths.

3. Imagine yourself lying on a beach on a beautiful, warm summer's day.

4. The beach is quiet and peaceful.

5. Feel the heat from the sun and the warmth of the sand.

6. See the waves as they gently glide onto the shore.

7. Notice their softness as they stroke the sand.

8. Continue to watch the waves as they gradually reach the shore.

9. See them get smaller and smaller, slower and slower, until they no longer grace the sand.

10. Look at the stillness of the crystal-clear water.

11. See the emptiness and serenity of the sea.

12. Breathe in slowly and deeply, hold for 5 seconds, and then slowly exhale. Do three more of these breaths.

13. Open your eyes.

EXERCISE 2: GENTLE MOTION

This relaxing exercise involves soft movements. With practice you will be able to carry it out as one flowing motion. The goal is to remain focused on your movement and postures and let all unwanted thoughts or feelings pass by.

1. Stand with your feet shoulder width apart and your arms relaxed by your sides.

2. Take a deep breath in and raise your arms up over your head.

3. As you exhale, gently lower your arms to the side and bring your right foot forward.

4. Take a deep breath in and slowly shift your weight onto your right leg and bring both arms out in front of you with your fingers extended and pointing forward.

5. As you exhale, return your right leg and arms back to the centre and bring your left foot forward.

6. Take a deep breath in and slowly shift your weight onto your left leg and bring both arms out in front of you with your fingers extended and pointing forward.

7. As you exhale, return your left leg and arms back to the centre.

8. Take a deep breath in and raise your arms up over your head.

9. As you exhale, slowly bend at the waist and reach down to the ground.

10. Take a deep breath in and gently bring your arms back up and reach up as high as you can.

11. As you exhale, bring your arms slowly back down to your sides.

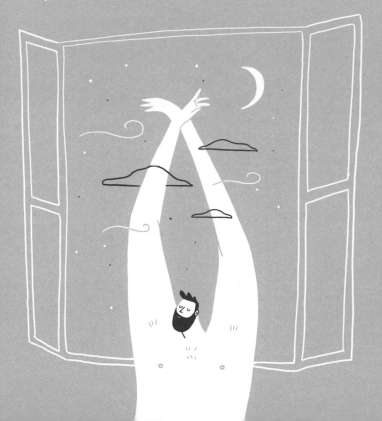

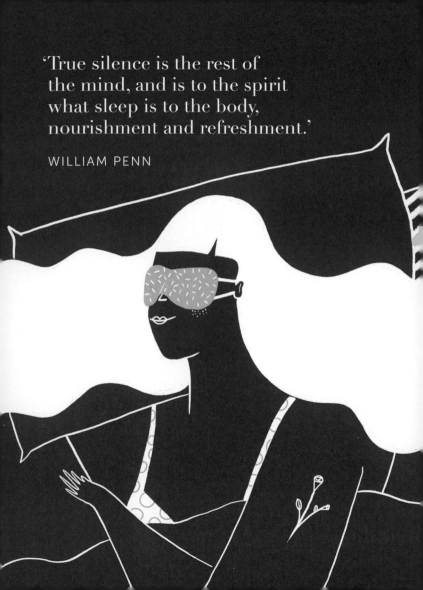

'True silence is the rest of the mind, and is to the spirit what sleep is to the body, nourishment and refreshment.'

WILLIAM PENN

THE BRAIN CHEMICALS THAT REGULATE SLEEP

The co-ordination of the sleep-wake cycle involves communication between different areas of the brain. The hypothalamus, thalamus, brainstem, basal forebrain and cerebral cortex are involved in the shift between sleep and wakefulness as well as the transitions between the sleep stages.

When the parts of the brain that control alertness are active, they inhibit the activity in the areas of the brain that are responsible for promoting sleep. Similarly, when the areas of the brain that produce sleep are most active, they inhibit the activity in areas of the brain that are responsible for promoting wakefulness.

The communication between the different parts of the brain that control sleep and wakefulness is carried out by hormones and neurotransmitters. The body's task of ensuring that those chemicals that promote sleep are not overwhelmed by those that stimulate alertness is an important one.

The key brain chemicals that regulate the sleep-wake cycle are:

SEROTONIN

Serotonin is often referred to as the 'happy hormone' because of its ability to elevate mood. It is produced in a part of the brainstem known as the raphe nuclei. In the sleep-wake cycle, serotonin promotes alertness and inhibits REM sleep. Low serotonin levels can cause frequent night-time waking.

MELATONIN

Melatonin is key to the circadian rhythm. Its presence makes us sleepy and its absence makes us alert. Melatonin is made from serotonin. It is also an important antioxidant, protecting our cells from free radicals (molecules that damage cells by altering their metabolism and division).

GAMMA-AMINOBUTYRIC ACID (GABA)

GABA is the most important inhibitory (calming) neurotransmitter in the brain. GABA decreases the activity of excitatory (stimulating) nerve cells. It is secreted from the ventrolateral preoptic nucleus (VLPO) of the hypothalamus, a key sleep-promoting area of the brain. It is thought that many conditions (including anxiety, insomnia and addiction) are related to reduced GABA activity.

ACETYLCHOLINE

Acetylcholine is a neurotransmitter that promotes REM sleep and is responsible for the rapid eye movement that is characteristic of this sleep stage. The acetylcholine nerve cells that regulate sleep are found in the basal forebrain and pons (part of the brainstem).

HISTAMINE

Histamine is a very powerful sleep-cycle regulator. It is produced in a part of the hypothalamus known as the tuberomammillary nucleus (TMN), a key wakefulness-promoting area of the brain. The level of histamine in the brain peaks during times of alertness and drops during sleep. It is also responsible for producing the symptoms that are commonly seen in an allergic reaction.

NOREPINEPHRINE

Norepinephrine is secreted towards the end of the night, which helps us wake up in the morning. It also supports the transition between NREM and REM sleep stages.

OREXIN/HYPOCRETIN

Orexin promotes alertness by stimulating histamine, norepinephrine and serotonin. It is produced in the hypothalamus. Reduced orexin function has been linked to narcolepsy.

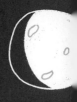

GLUTAMATE

Glutamate is the most important excitatory neurotransmitter in the brain. Surprisingly, it is made from GABA. Glutamate promotes alertness by stimulating the activity of orexin.

CORTISOL

Cortisol is a wakefulness-promoting hormone that is made in the adrenal glands and released in response to stress. Normally, its level is highest in the morning and lowest during the night.

CORTICOTROPIN-RELEASING HORMONE (CRH)

CRH is secreted by the paraventricular nucleus of the hypothalamus during stress. CRH stimulates wakefulness and reduces the amount of time spent in REM sleep.

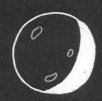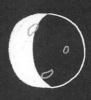

ADRENOCORTICOTROPIC HORMONE (ACTH)

The secretion of ACTH is triggered by CRH. ACTH stimulates the release of cortisol. ACTH increases alertness and its level is highest in the morning.

GROWTH HORMONE-RELEASING HORMONE (GHRH)

GHRH increases the duration and depth of NREM sleep. Its main role in the body is triggering the release of growth hormone from the anterior pituitary gland.

GLYCINE

Glycine is an amino acid that acts as a neurotransmitter. It is calming and helps to trigger sleep by dropping body temperature at night. Glycine is also responsible for producing the absence of muscle tone that occurs during REM sleep.

DOPAMINE

Dopamine is an important wakefulness promoter. It decreases the production of melatonin towards the end of the night. In addition, new research is suggesting that dopamine may be important in establishing REM sleep and helping to produce muscle immobility.

NEUROPEPTIDE S

Neuropeptide S promotes alertness and stimulates the release of dopamine. It also plays a role in reducing feelings of anxiety during stressful situations.

NEUROPEPTIDE Y

Neuropeptide Y is a neurotransmitter that promotes sleep by inhibiting the release of CRH. Neuropeptide Y is also able to shift the timing of the circadian clock.

ADENOSINE

Adenosine is an important sleep-wake cycle regulator. The level of adenosine increases throughout the day and peaks at night. Sleep pressure builds with increasing adenosine. Adenosine acts to promote brain relaxation and encourage NREM sleep. Caffeine exerts its stimulating effect by blocking the action of adenosine.

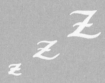

YAWNING: ONE OF LIFE'S GREAT MYSTERIES

We have all been yawning since the beginning of time. Yet surprisingly, we know very little about it. We do know that we yawn when we are tired. This may be because yawns are triggered by certain brain chemicals that encourage sleep, including glycine. Yawning is also initiated by alertness-promoting chemicals like serotonin, dopamine and ACTH. This is why we often yawn in the morning.

There are a number of theories as to why we yawn. Some researchers suggested that yawning acts as a reflex to increase the intake of oxygen when levels are low. Others believe that yawning strengthens and protects the lungs. It has also been proposed that yawning cools the brain during times of overactivity.

A well-known characteristic of yawning is that it is contagious. No one knows exactly why this is the case but some of the proposed ideas include: empathy, imitation, age (older people are less likely to experience contagious yawning), an increased need for oxygen when a nearby person takes too much, and genetics.

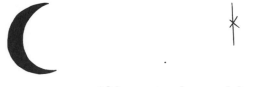

'Sleep is the golden
chain that ties health and
our bodies together.'

THOMAS DEKKER

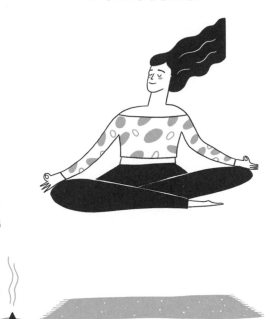

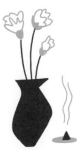

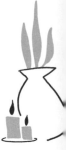

SLEEP NOURISHES THE MIND AND THE BODY

There is no doubt that humans need sleep. When we are deprived of it, our bodies do whatever is in their means to obtain it. Yet, when it comes to explaining exactly why we sleep, there is still much that is unknown. Experts have put forward several theories, most of which have some very convincing evidence. However, each one on its own does not tell the whole story. The answer is likely found in a combination of these theories.

What we do know for certain is that sleep has many health benefits and is one of nature's best medicines for prevention. Just as the food we eat provides us with nutrients that feed and support our tissues and organs, sleep provides us a time for growth, replenishment and rejuvenation.

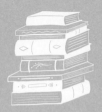

WHY DO WE SLEEP?

THE THEORY OF ENERGY CONSERVATION

This is also known as the evolutionary theory or the adaptive theory. It is based on the idea that sleep reduces a person's need to expend energy during times when they are less likely to find food. Our metabolism decreases at night so there is some merit to this theory.

THE THEORY OF INACTIVITY

The idea here is that being inactive at night makes a person less likely to be injured or attacked by predators. This theory has been questioned because inactivity (sleep) can make a person more vulnerable to predatory attack.

THE THEORY OF RESTORATION

This theory states that sleep provides a time for the body to repair itself. There is substantial evidence supporting this as we know that the body's repair and restore mechanisms are hard at work while we sleep. Hormone release and cell repair during sleep have been demonstrated.

THE THEORY OF BRAIN PLASTICITY

The idea here is that sleep is necessary for the growth and development of the brain. This is true, as we know that neuronal connections are established and strengthened while we sleep. Evidence for the ability to retain information during sleep has been found.

THE THEORY OF DETOXIFICATION

This theory says that sleep is a time for the body to rid itself of impurities. We know that neurotoxins are removed from the brain while we sleep, including β-amyloid which has been found to accumulate in the brains of those with Alzheimer's disease. It has also been shown that the activity of glutathione peroxidase (an enzyme that protects our cells from damage) in the brain is higher at night.

SLEEP AND MEMORY

We learn new information and perform complex tasks every day. How is this information retained? How are we able to remember the steps of a task we performed so we can repeat the procedure in the future? Currently, it is thought that much of this remarkable feat is carried out in the hippocampus and other cortical regions of the brain while we sleep.

The procedure by which the brain integrates new memories into its established network is known as memory consolidation. In the brain, this occurs when the neurons within a group fire together enough times to create a permanent association with one another. Existing connections between neurons are also strengthened during the process.

Currently, it is thought that memories related to facts and events (known as declarative memories) are consolidated during delta sleep. In contrast, emotional memories and technical (how to do things) memories appear to be consolidated during REM sleep.

Sleep is so important to the establishment of new memories because it is a time of mental relaxation and unbiased thinking. While we sleep we are not receiving any new facts, learning to perform any new tasks or engaged in any new experiences. Therefore, our daytime occurrences can enter into the brain's permanent collection unimpeded. In addition, the closer to bedtime that a new procedure is learned or new information is received, the less likely it is to be forgotten or distorted and the more likely it is to become an accurate memory.

THE REWARDS WE REAP FROM A GOOD NIGHT'S SLEEP

TISSUE GROWTH AND REPAIR

While we sleep, growth hormone is secreted from the anterior pituitary. Growth hormone has a number of important roles, including triggering the secretion of another hormone known as insulin-like growth factor-1 (IGF-1) from the liver and elsewhere. IGF-1 stimulates muscle growth and repair and bone growth. Growth hormone also promotes protein synthesis and fat breakdown and normalizes blood sugar levels.

A HEALTHY IMMUNE SYSTEM

Sleep reduces inflammation by keeping the levels of pro-inflammatory cytokines, like IL-1β and TNF-α (see page 23), in check. Sleep enhances the body's ability to fight off infections and is protective against the development of autoimmune conditions. Sleep also assists in the development of immunological memory, which is the ability of the immune system to quickly fight off an invader that it has already encountered in the past.

A HEALTHY MIND

Sleep promotes the establishment of proper neuronal connections. Sleep also supports the formation of myelin, a protective coating around nerve cells. Studies on the effects of sleep deprivation have shown that sleep is essential for proper cognitive functioning. Sleep promotes attention and alertness. Those who sleep well are less likely to have accidents or make mistakes. Sleep is necessary for learning new information and accessing previously acquired information. Sleep enhances the ability to reason and make decisions. We also tend to feel happier, more energetic and less anxious following deep and restful sleep.

IMPROVED PHYSICAL HEALTH

Sleep enhances endurance and athletic performance. Sleep protects against muscle aches, joint pain and migraine headaches. Those who are sleep-deprived tend to be more sensitive to pain and are more likely to experience a worsening of conditions, such as rheumatoid arthritis and osteoarthritis.

A HEALTHY WAISTLINE

Sleep controls appetite and reduces cravings for unhealthy foods. Lack of sleep increases the level of the hormone ghrelin, which stimulates appetite. Sleep also keeps cortisol levels at bay. Elevated cortisol increases body fat, especially around the belly.

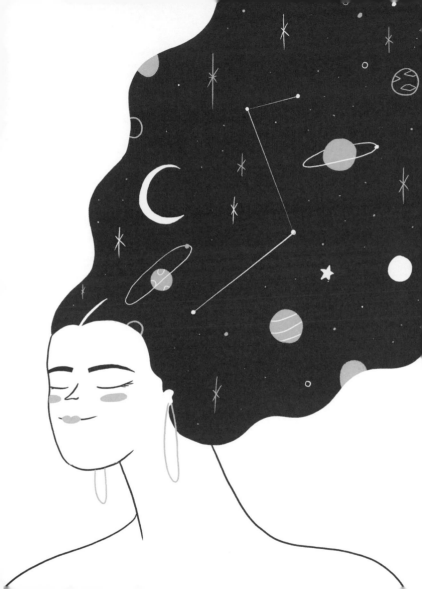

BALANCED HORMONES

Sleep is essential for hormone balance. Proper control of the amounts of insulin and glucagon (hormones that regulate blood sugar levels) is reliant on sufficient sleep. Sleep protects against insulin resistance and keeps blood sugar levels at bay. Changes in metabolism due to alterations in thyroid hormone levels has been observed in those who experience sleep loss. Sleep also regulates the levels of the sex hormones, including oestrogen and testosterone. Sex hormone imbalances can cause low libido, fatigue, mood swings, hair loss, skin changes, weight gain, night sweats and infertility.

SLEEP IS YOUR BEST BEAUTY TREATMENT

Sleep not only heals you on the inside, it also promotes a healthy and youthful appearance on the outside. During sleep, the collagen matrix is strengthened and the circulation to the skin is enhanced. Your skin will become more hydrated and fine lines and wrinkles will reduce. Getting the right amount of sleep will keep your hair smooth and lustrous. It can also reduce your risk of experiencing hair loss.

I'M NOT A NIGHT-SLEEPER. HOW DO I ENJOY THESE HEALTH BENEFITS?

For a variety of reasons, many of us are not able to obtain the recommended hours of night-time slumber. Whether we are travelling across time zones, working night shifts, working alternating shifts or caring for an infant during the night, our circumstances may not allow us to have a continuous period of sleep at an ideal time. The best way to stay alert and healthy is to sleep whenever possible for as long as possible. Keeping a consistent schedule is also important. Limiting travel distances and shift rotations can help to ensure that sleep and wake times are regular. Exposure to full-spectrum lighting while working at night can help to adjust your circadian clock.

Reaping the rewards of a healthy sleep-wake cycle also involves taking care of yourself during the 'wake' component. Having a loved one or close friend assist with the shopping, childcare or any other tasks or responsibilities you may have can be very beneficial. Allotting time to socialize, exercise and take part in hobbies and activities you enjoy will not only help to build up sleep pressure but will also enhance your overall feelings of emotional and physical wellbeing.

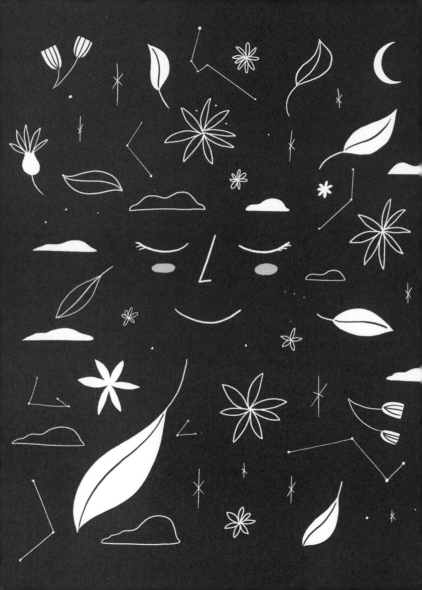

WHAT'S IN A DREAM?

The act of dreaming and the analysis of dreams have been a source of interest since the beginning of humanity. Dreams can be extraordinarily vivid or extremely vague. They can be filled with joyful images or frightening situations. Dreams can be straightforward and direct or unclear and mystifying. Throughout history philosophers and scientists have been baffled by dreams. To this day, dreams continue to be a source of mystery and their content a source of wonder.

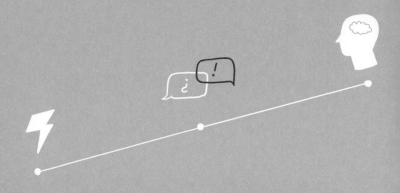

THE DREAM TIMELINE

Beliefs and theories regarding the purpose and meaning of dreams have evolved over time.

A SUPERNATURAL OCCURRENCE

Early civilizations believed that dreams contained prophetic messages from the Gods. It was common practice to have dreams interpreted by a priest or diviner. The information provided in the dreams was used to make decisions and guide daily life. When bad dreams occurred, they were not discussed as this would make them more likely to come true. The ancient Egyptians practised dream incubation, in which they performed rituals in order to evoke helpful dreams that could provide answers to questions or solutions to problems. The overall belief was that dreams are a passive experience and their content is divine in origin.

DREAMS ORIGINATE IN THE MIND

In the 5th century BC academics began to question the origin of dreams. The Greek philosopher Heraclitus believed that the content of dreams comes from the mind. Aristotle did not believe that dreams were divine in origin and thought that if a dream happened to predict a future event, it was merely a coincidence.

DREAMS ARE A REFLECTION OF THE MIND

During the Renaissance period between the 14th and 17th centuries there was a growing interest in identifying the source of dreams. Dream interpretation was relatively uncommon. Physicians began to explore the relationship between dreams and health. The Italian physician Girolamo Cardano believed that there was a connection between a person's dream and their emotional state.

MODERN THEORIES OF DREAMING

WISH FULFILLMENT THEORY

In the early 20th century, neurologist Sigmund Freud developed the theory that dreams serve the purpose of wish fulfillment. They occur as a result of the subconscious mind trying to solve a conflict or satisfy a desire. He identified two different types of dream content: the thoughts and images contained within the dream and their unconscious meaning. Freud also brought dream interpretation back into prominence.

ACTIVATION-SYNTHESIS THEORY

This theory was proposed by John Allan Hobson and Robert McCarley in 1977. It suggests that dreams are the result of random signals generated by the brain during REM sleep, and promotes the idea that during REM sleep, areas of the brainstem become active. This activity then stimulates the limbic system, which is the part of the brain that controls emotion and memory. Dreams are thought to result from the activity in these areas.

REVERSE LEARNING THEORY

This theory was proposed by Francis Crick and Graeme Mitchison in 1983. It suggests that dreaming is a time when the brain eliminates what it doesn't need. The brain acquires a great deal of information during waking hours. During REM sleep the brain sorts through this data, looking for unwanted neuronal connections which contain incorrect memories or undesirable information. Dreaming is a time when these unwanted neuronal connections are removed.

CONTINUAL-ACTIVATION THEORY

This theory was proposed by Jie Zhang in 2004. It states that dreams occur as a by-product of the transfer of memories from a temporary hold to long-term storage. Zhang believes that there are two types of dreams, those that are produced when declarative memories are transferred and those that are produced when technical memories are transferred.

MEMORY CONSOLIDATION THEORY

Building upon the Continual-activation Theory, this one posits the idea that dreams happen as a result of the 'reactivation' of memories that occurs during their consolidation.

EVOLUTIONARY THEORY

This theory suggests that dreams serve the purpose of enhancing the survival of our species. Dreams provide us with insight and help us solve problems, formulate ideas and develop new skills. Antti Revonsuo, a neuroscientist, believes that nightmares also serve an evolutionary purpose. He proposes that they provide us with an opportunity to practise navigating dangerous situations. This will in turn prepare us and increase our chances of survival should we encounter a threat.

CONTEMPORARY THEORY

This theory sees dreaming as a type of therapy. Dreams are guided by our emotions and what we experience in our day-to-day lives. The purpose of dreaming is to help us make connections based on our emotions. Dreams also serve to lessen the effects of strong emotions and negative experiences. The vividness and intensity of a dream is determined by the emotional state of the dreamer.

WHAT DO OUR DREAMS TRULY MEAN?

At one time or another, you have likely found yourself pondering over the meaning of a dream that you've had. The dream may have centered around a discussion at the office, an argument with your partner, a meal at your favourite restaurant or an afternoon at the shops. There is also the chance that your dream may have had no centre of focus. It could have consisted of images of the dog you had as a child and your son eating his first ice cream cone. What is the inherent message? What are we to gain from this?

As we know from the many theories, dreams can be any number of things. They could be revealing our deepest desires or be the result of random nerve firings. When seeking to understand dreams it is best to look at them in two respects: circumstance and frequency.

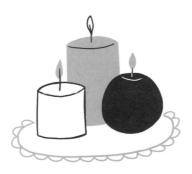

THE CIRCUMSTANCE OF A DREAM

- Does the content of the dream display, or bring attention to, a situation that is affecting my life in the present?

- Does the content of the dream display, or bring attention to, a situation that affected me in the past?

- Does the content of the dream invoke strong emotions, either during the dream or after I wake up?

THE FREQUENCY OF A DREAM

- Does any aspect of the content of this dream appear familiar to me?

- Have I had this exact dream before?

There is evidence suggesting that dreams can be a reflection of our waking lives, particularly those aspects that are joyous or worrisome. If you find that the circumstance of a dream is such that it pertains to a facet of your life that is challenging, you may need to look at ways to manage, if not overcome, your obstacle. Similarly, a recurring theme may direct you to a situation in your life that needs your attention.

LUCID DREAMING

A lucid dream is one in which a person is aware that they are dreaming. Sometimes, the dreamer is able to control the story, thoughts or images within the dream. Lucid dreaming can have a positive impact on daily life. The dreamer may be able to solve problems or participate in an enjoyable hobby or activity in the dream. This can lead to reduced stress and an increased sense of wellbeing while the person is awake. Many lucid dreamers report an ability to achieve a higher level of consciousness during waking life. Lucid dreaming may also help to bring about a sense of inner peace and spiritual enlightenment.

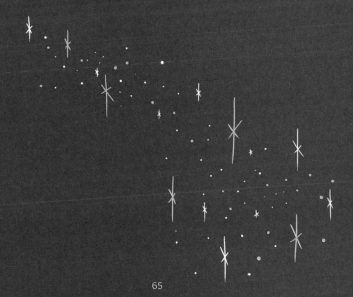

WHEN SLEEP IS DISRUPTED

We know that getting an average of 6–8 hours of sleep per night is recommended for most adults, but what happens if this is not achievable? Sleeping difficulties are not uncommon. In fact, if you ask most people, they will likely tell you that they have experienced at least a night or two of little or no sleep. It is not unusual for stress or worry to keep us up now and then. However, sleep disruption can have a number of causes, other than an upcoming deadline or a big presentation first thing in the morning.

ARTIFICIAL LIGHTING

Artificial light emitted from televisions, computers, tablets, mobile phones and energy-saving lightbulbs is rich in blue light. Blue light can suppress the secretion of melatonin.

BED PARTNER

A person who snores, frequently moves their legs or tosses and turns while they sleep can make falling asleep and staying asleep very difficult for their bed partner.

CAFFEINE

Caffeine acts as a sleep disruptor by blocking the action of adenosine. It also promotes the release of histamine, cortisol and adrenaline. Caffeine is found in coffee, tea

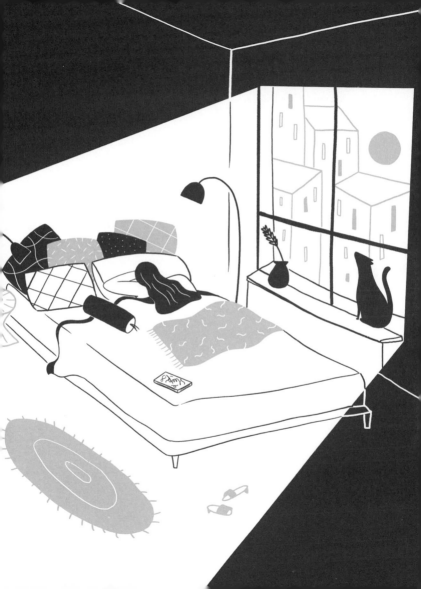

(black, green, white and oolong), guarana, mate, energy drinks, chocolate, kola nut and cola drinks.

CHANGING SCHEDULES

Humans are known to be creatures of habit. Our circadian clocks thrive on a set routine. Travel between time zones and rotating work shifts can alter the sleep-wake cycle. Those who experience frequent schedule changes often report difficulty falling asleep and decreased sleep quality.

CITY LIFE AND THE NOISY NEIGHBOUR

Where we live can certainly dictate how easy it will be to nod off. A city full of bright lights and loud traffic can make a good night's sleep very difficult to achieve. Also, your neighbour can play a big part in determining your sleep schedule. Living adjacent to those who enjoy cinema-like sound on their televisions or those who frequently host social gatherings that extend well into the night could put a damper on your sleep plans.

CONFLICT

The old saying 'never go to bed angry' certainly has merit. Not only can anger keep you tossing and turning, but research has shown that sleep can store negative memories in such a way that they become harder to suppress or eliminate in the future. This can lead to resentment, further conflict and continued sleep loss.

FOODS AND ADDITIVES

Heavily sweetened foods can reduce the secretion of melatonin and stimulate the release of hormones that promote alertness. Additives such as monosodium glutamate (MSG), artificial food colourings, fat stabilizers (e.g. butylated hydroxyanisole (BHA) and butylated hydroxytoluene (BHT)) and benzoates have been linked to hyperactivity and sleep loss.

GRIEF

A life event that brings us heartache and sorrow can make a good night's sleep very hard to come by. The effects of grief on the sleep-wake cycle and other body systems are most pronounced in the first three months following the loss. Grief triggers the stress response and increases the level of cortisol, resulting in greater alertness and frequent waking. Those who have experienced loss often have difficulty falling asleep and spend less time in the deeper sleep stages once they drift off. Increased inflammation, heart rate and blood pressure can also occur during the initial stages of grief.

ILLNESS

Several health conditions produce difficulty falling asleep or fragmented sleep. Digestive ailments, diabetes, heart disease, kidney disease, anxiety, depression, bipolar disorder, schizophrenia, brain injury, neurological conditions, asthma, hyperthyroidism and cancer can all negatively affect sleep.

LONG-STANDING STRESS OR WORRY

Our bodies are equipped to handle a moderate amount of stress. Some people actually thrive and perform at their peak in high-pressure situations. However, when there is too much stress, or the stress is prolonged, the body's stress management system becomes overworked. This leads to high amounts of cortisol and adrenaline causing sleeping difficulties, weight gain, a reduced ability to fight infections, thyroid hormone imbalances, depression, weak bones and poor blood sugar control. If this situation persists, the outcome is a depletion of the body's reserves and burnout. This leads to mental and physical exhaustion and an increased susceptibility to disease.

LOW CARBOHYDRATE DIET

The hormone melatonin is synthesized from serotonin, which in turn is made from the amino acid tryptophan. Unfortunately, tryptophan has to compete with other amino acids to enter the brain because they use the same transport system. Luckily, tryptophan is able to beat out the competition by the presence of insulin, which is a hormone released from the pancreas following the consumption of carbohydrates. Therefore, eating unrefined carbohydrates, such as fruits, vegetables and wholegrains can help get the tryptophan to where it needs to be to produce melatonin.

MEDICATIONS

Common medications such as beta blockers (e.g. atenolol, propranolol), corticosteroids (e.g. prednisolone, hydrocortisone), decongestants (e.g. pseudoephedrine, phenylephrine), statins (e.g. atorvastatin, simvastatin) and selective serotonin reuptake inhibitors (e.g. escitalopram, dapoxetine) can reduce the time spent in REM sleep, NREM sleep or both.

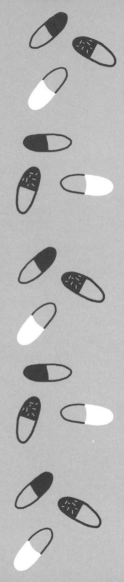

MOTHER NATURE

Sometimes factors that are not in our control can affect our sleep. Genetics can make a person more prone to develop a sleep disorder or another type of condition that produces sleep loss as a symptom. Gender can also play a role in determining how soundly we sleep. Women often report more sleep problems than men. There are also gender-based differences in the prevalence of certain sleep disorders. Women are more likely to suffer from insomnia while men are more likely to lose sleep as a result of sleep-disordered breathing. Hormonal changes that occur in life, such as during menses, menopause and andropause, often lead to sleep disruption. Pregnancy can produce sleep loss due to nausea, heartburn, back pain, leg cramps and intense dreams.

PAIN

Any disorder that causes pain can lead to sleep disruption. Common conditions include muscle strain, ligament sprain, osteoarthritis, headache, fibromyalgia, viral illness (like the flu) and hypothyroidism. In turn, a lack of sleep can make a painful condition worse.

SLEEP-DISORDERED BREATHING

This refers to atypical breathing patterns during sleep. Common types of sleep-disordered breathing are sleep apnoea and sleep-related hypoventilation. Those who suffer from sleep-disordered breathing experience frequent waking and unrefreshing sleep.

UNCOMFORTABLE MATTRESS OR PILLOW

An old or soft mattress that does not offer support or a fluffy pillow that leaves your neck feeling stiff can lead to many nights of tossing and turning.

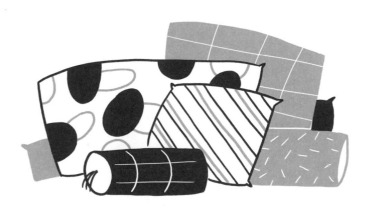

CONSEQUENCES OF LONG-TERM SLEEP LOSS

Most of us know what it feels like to be sleep-deprived. We can be irritable, forgetful and have difficulty concentrating. Our muscles may be sore, our eyes bloodshot and we may feel fatigued or have a general sense of malaise. The symptoms of short-term sleep loss vary from person to person. One person may be unfazed by a couple of late nights and early mornings, while another may be slumped at their desk enduring continuous episodes of yawning.

When we experience long-term sleep loss, our symptoms can become far more pronounced. Our risk of developing a number of chronic diseases also increases. Long-standing sleep deprivation has been associated with an increased likelihood of developing:

- Obesity
- Type 2 diabetes
- High blood pressure
- Heart disease
- Cancer
- Alzheimer's disease
- Stomach ulcers
- Irritable bowel syndrome
- Inflammatory bowel disease
- Anxiety
- Depression

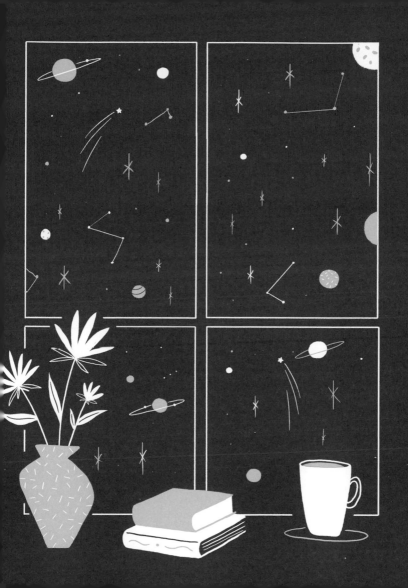

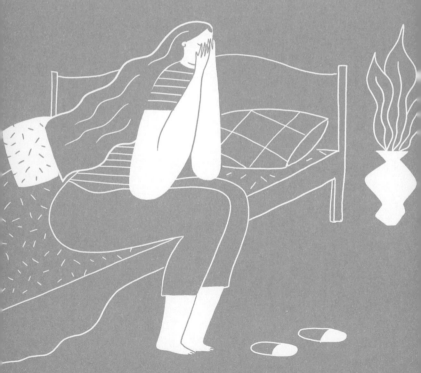

'Insomnia is a gross feeder.
It will nourish itself on any
kind of thinking, including
thinking about not thinking.'

CLIFTON FADIMAN

WHAT IS INSOMNIA?

At present, there are about 60 classified sleep disorders. They all vary in how significantly they impact sleep and in their ability to produce daytime symptoms. The most common sleep disorder is insomnia.

Insomnia refers to difficulty falling asleep, difficulty staying asleep and/or early morning awakening. The causes of insomnia are numerous and include stress, worry, sadness, pain, problems with the sleep environment, unhealthy daytime and bedtime habits, psychological or physical illness and medications.

Those who suffer from insomnia experience non-refreshing sleep and symptoms of daytime impairment that include: tiredness, low energy, irritability, poor concentration and impaired academic, social, occupational or behavioural functioning. Insomnia affects about one-third of the UK population.

CATEGORIES OF INSOMNIA

	Short-term insomnia disorder	Chronic insomnia disorder	Other insomnia disorder
Duration	Sleeping difficulty that lasts less than 3 months	Sleeping difficulty that occurs at least 3 times per week for 3 months or more	Those who experience typical insomnia features (sleeping difficulty, ample sleep opportunity and daytime dysfunction), but do not meet the full criteria for either short-term insomnia disorder or chronic insomnia disorder
Additional criteria needed for the diagnosis	• The sleeping difficulty occurs despite ample opportunity for sleep • The sleeping difficulty is not better explained by another sleep disorder • The sleeping difficulty is accompanied by at least one symptom of daytime impairment		

HOW IS INSOMNIA DETECTED?

- Information provided by the insomnia-sufferer themselves, their bed partner and/or their caregiver.

- Findings from a physical examination.

- Questionnaires such as the Epworth Sleepiness Scale and the Insomnia Severity Index.

- Polysomnography: a sleep study that includes the assessment of brain waves (using an EEG), eye movements (using an EOG), muscle action (using an electromyogram (EMG)), heart rhythm (using an electrocardiogram (ECG or EKG)), blood oxygen levels (using a pulse oximeter) and breathing (using an air flow transducer).

- Actigraphy: a study in which a person wears a sensor that assesses their sleep patterns. This is often used to rule out the presence of another sleep disorder.

- Blood tests or other diagnostic testing. This can help determine if another condition is causing the insomnia.

IF IT ISN'T INSOMNIA, WHAT ELSE COULD IT BE?

Although insomnia is fairly common, there are many other sleep disorders that could be keeping you awake at night. Some of the more prevalent ones are:

SLEEP APNOEA

Sleep apnoea is a common sleep-related breathing disorder in which brief interruptions in breathing occur during sleep. The sufferer experiences daytime tiredness and is often unaware of the pauses in breathing. Sleep apnoea is diagnosed by polysomnography.

There are two main types of sleep apnoea:

1. OBSTRUCTIVE SLEEP APNOEA SYNDROMES: These are the most common type. They occur when the soft tissue in the back of the throat relaxes during sleep and blocks the airway. Snoring is a common symptom of obstructive sleep apnoea. Risk factors for the development of obstructive sleep apnoea syndromes include high blood pressure, obesity, allergies, asthma, hypothyroidism and smoking.

2. CENTRAL SLEEP APNOEA SYNDROMES:
These are far less common. They involve the central nervous system and occur when the brain fails to tell your muscles to breathe. Risk factors for the development of central sleep apnoea syndromes include congestive heart failure, stroke, brain tumour, high altitude and the use of opiates.

DELAYED SLEEP-WAKE PHASE DISORDER (DSWPD)

This is a disruption of the circadian rhythm causing a person to be unable to fall asleep until the early hours of the morning, usually between 2am and 6am. Those who have the condition are often referred to as 'extreme night owls'. They have difficulty waking up for work or school and experience excessive daytime sleepiness. The cause of DSWPD is thought to be genetic and the diagnosis is confirmed by actigraphy. DSWPD is a type of circadian rhythm sleep-wake disorder, a group of sleep disorders that involve alterations in the circadian clock.

RESTLESS LEGS SYNDROME (RLS)

This is a sleep-related movement disorder in which a person experiences discomfort in the legs while at rest at night. The discomfort is relieved with movement and often results in sleeping difficulty at night. The possible causes of restless legs syndrome include genetics, pregnancy, low dopamine levels, iron deficiency, kidney failure or prolonged immobility. The existence of the condition is identified by the suggested immobilization test, during which you will be asked to lie down in an attempt to provoke the symptoms of restless legs syndrome.

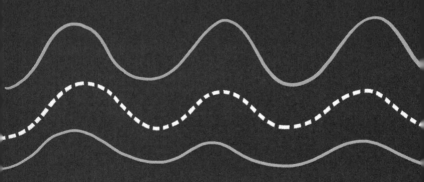

NARCOLEPSY

Narcolepsy involves uncontrollable episodes of falling asleep during the daytime or excessive daytime sleepiness for at least three months. It is a type of central disorder of hypersomnolence, which is a group of sleep disorders that involve the inability to stay awake or alert during the day. Other symptoms include cataplexy (sudden episodes of temporary muscle weakness), sleep paralysis (a brief inability to move or speak when falling asleep or while waking up) and sleeping difficulties at night. The causes of narcolepsy are genetics, illness, the destruction of orexin-producing neurons by the body's immune system, brain injury or a brain tumour. Narcolepsy is diagnosed by polysomnography and the multiple sleep latency test which will determine how quickly you are able to fall asleep during the day and how soon you enter REM sleep.

There are two types of narcolepsy:

- NARCOLEPSY TYPE 1:
  This type is characterized by cataplexy, drifting off quickly and entering REM soon after falling asleep and/or low levels of orexin-A.

- NARCOLEPSY TYPE 2:
  Those with narcolepsy type 2 do not suffer from cataplexy nor do they have very low levels of orexin-A. They do drift off quickly and enter REM soon after falling asleep.

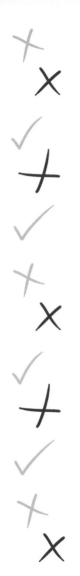

TRUE OR FALSE?

There are beliefs about sleep that many of us have likely heard. Although some are based on fact, many are rooted in fiction. Those that are untrue can make us worry unnecessarily or give us unrealistic expectations. When it comes to sleep it can often be difficult to discern between what is true and what is false.

'INSOMNIA WILL ALWAYS RESOLVE ON ITS OWN': **FALSE**

Sometimes a traumatic situation or an upcoming stressful event can lead to a brief period of insomnia that subsides when the situation has resolved, or the event has passed. However, this is not always the case. The effects of both emotional and physical trauma can last for years. Therefore, the insomnia could persist or recur from time to time.

Another reason that insomnia tends to linger is that it is often associated with a particular underlying issue, be it an illness or a certain medication. Therefore, unless the problem that is contributing to the insomnia is addressed, the sleeping difficulties will continue indefinitely.

'ADULTS MUST GET BETWEEN 6 AND 8 HOURS OF SLEEP EVERY NIGHT': FALSE

Although this is considered the ideal amount of sleep, there are those who require more and those who can make do with less. The best amount of sleep is that which allows you to wake up feeling refreshed and enables you to function optimally throughout the day.

'IF I SLEEP POORLY I SHOULD TAKE IT EASY THE FOLLOWING DAY': FALSE

Resting or taking it easy during the day does very little to grow your sleep pressure. If you have a night of poor sleep, you should stick to your schedule as much as possible the next day. Remaining as active as you can will ensure that you will be sleep-ready when your head hits the pillow.

'IF I HAVE INSOMNIA I MUST BE ANXIOUS': **FALSE**

Although insomnia can occur in cases of anxiety, a person does not have to be anxious to experience insomnia. Poor sleep can occur alongside several different conditions, both physical and psychological. For example, chronic pain can certainly produce insomnia, with or without accompanying anxiety. Therefore, if you are experiencing insomnia you may, or may not, suffer from anxiety.

'MOST OF OUR DREAMS ARE FORGOTTEN SHORTLY AFTER WAKING': **TRUE**

It is believed that 90 per cent of what we dreamt about will be forgotten 10 minutes after waking. This may be the result of the brain's housekeeping, during which it eliminates what it feels it doesn't need. Another possibility is that our brains like to remember thoughts that are structured, and oftentimes dreams consist of scattered or unorganized thoughts and images.

Due to the demands of daily life, many of us wake up to the sound of an alarm rather than gradually with the emergence of daylight and sound of chirping birds. The noise of the alarm often puts us in a temporary state of confusion and, once it dissipates, we are left mentally scanning our to-do lists and planning our tasks for the day. This will likely not leave our brains with enough power for dream recollection.

'WE ONLY DREAM DURING THE REM SLEEP STAGE': **FALSE**

This is a very popular myth. In actuality, about 80–90 per cent of our dreaming occurs during REM sleep and 10–20 per cent occurs in NREM sleep. REM dreams tend to be more vivid, so they are the ones we are inclined to remember when we wake. REM dreams are also more likely than NREM dreams to be aggressive, motivated and contain negative interactions and emotions. NREM dreams tend to have more positive interactions and cheerful emotions.

'SHORT-TERM INSOMNIA IS MORE COMMON THAN CHRONIC INSOMNIA': **TRUE**

Short-term insomnia disorder affects about 25 per cent of the adult population while chronic insomnia disorder afflicts 10 per cent of the population.

'I SHOULD DRIFT OFF AS SOON AS MY HEAD HITS THE PILLOW': **FALSE**

It takes up to 15 minutes for the average person to fall asleep. If you fall asleep the moment you lie down, it may be a sign that you are sleep-deprived. Conversely, if it takes you far longer to fall asleep you may be suffering from a sleep disorder.

'SLEEPING PILLS ARE THE ONLY AVAILABLE TREATMENT FOR INSOMNIA': **FALSE**

This is certainly a myth. Although medications continue to be the most common treatment, their effectiveness and safety have come into question in recent years. Cognitive behavioural therapy (CBT) has been found to be an effective tool in the management of insomnia. Stress management, regular physical activity and a healthy diet can also help to promote a good night's sleep.

'IT IS NORMAL TO BE GROGGY IN THE MORNING': **TRUE**

Grogginess is very common, particularly after your alarm pulls you abruptly out of sleep. This grogginess, known as sleep inertia, can last anywhere from a few minutes to 4 hours after waking. For most people, this tiredness persists for 15–30 minutes. Problems arise if we have to perform a complex mental or physical task while experiencing sleep inertia.

Sleep deprivation can make grogginess worse. This is because adenosine levels are still high when you wake up, which causes sleepiness. Being woken from stage 3 of sleep produces more detrimental sleep inertia than being roused during the lighter sleep stages. Sleep inertia can be worse after napping, particularly following an afternoon nap that is longer than 30 minutes.

'SNORING ALWAYS INDICATES A BREATHING DISORDER': **FALSE**

Although snoring is common in those who have sleep apnoea, not everyone who snores has the disorder. Snoring is the loud sound that occurs when the air that you breathe makes the relaxed tissues at the back of your throat vibrate. Snoring has several possible causes including allergies, a cold, obesity, sleeping on your back, pregnancy, drinking alcohol, sleep loss, enlarged tonsils and a deviated nasal septum.

'ALCOHOL IS AN EFFECTIVE SLEEP AID': **FALSE**

Historically, people have used alcohol to help them nod off. Although alcohol can reduce the time it takes to fall asleep, it causes frequent waking, increases body temperature and decreases melatonin. Using alcohol as a sleep aid can increase the risk of sleepwalking and sleep apnoea. Regular use can lead to dependence.

'WAKING UP FOR A FEW MINUTES DURING THE NIGHT IS HARMLESS': **FALSE**

Studies have shown that those who wake up during the night, but who sleep for a full 7–8 hours, can feel just as tired in the morning as those who sleep no more than 4–5 hours. Therefore, if you are waking up during the night (other than for work or to comfort or feed a crying infant) you should look into the reason why.

'I WILL NEED LESS SLEEP AS I GET OLDER': **FALSE**

Many people tend to wake more frequently as they age. Also, the amount of time spent in the deeper stages of sleep decreases with age. This may make an older person feel groggy and unrefreshed in the morning. That being said, all adults require the same number of hours of sleep regardless of age. Therefore, daytime napping is quite common for the aging adult in order to make up for lost, or light, sleep during the night.

'CHILDREN DON'T GET INSOMNIA': **FALSE**

If you are a parent or work with children, you probably know this to be untrue. About 25 per cent of children experience insomnia at one time or another. Unlike adults, children usually don't realize that they have trouble sleeping until they begin to notice daytime effects, such as drowsiness and difficulty concentrating.

Nightmares and bed-wetting are common in children and may (but not always) cause insomnia. Children experience stress and worry just like adults do. Separation anxiety, bullying or the 'end of summer blues' (nervous anticipation about the forthcoming school year) are just a few of the many sources of stress that can keep a child from getting the sleep that they need.

Poor night-time habits, such as too much screen time before bed, can contribute to insomnia. The processed foods that are marketed to children are often rich in refined sugar and low in essential nutrients, which can cause sleep disruption.

Childhood insomnia, whether it lasts one night or one year, should always be investigated and treated. If left untreated, insomnia in children tends to recur. Long-standing insomnia can negatively affect a child's academic performance, strain friendships and increase the likelihood of developing chronic conditions like diabetes and heart disease later in life.

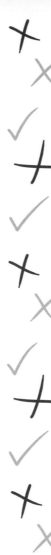

A RETURN TO RESTFUL SLEEP

When it comes to the treatment of sleep disorders there are a number of options. The frequency and types of therapies used will depend on your symptoms, the nature of the sleep problem and the severity of the condition.

Treatments used for a number of sleep disorders may be similar because the desired outcomes are usually to enhance the depth and duration of sleep and to reduce the occurrence of sleepiness or wakefulness at inappropriate times.

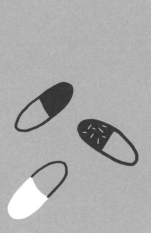

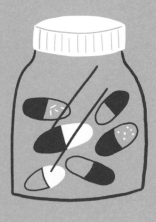

MEDICATIONS

Medications are often the first treatment given for sleep loss.

FOR INSOMNIA

Over-the-counter medications, such as diphenhydramine and doxylamine block wakefulness-promoting histamine. Prescription medications used to produce sedation include lorazepam, diazepam, temazepam, zaleplon, zolpidem, eszopiclone. A new class of medicines that block orexin can be helpful in the treatment of insomnia. Examples are suvorexant and lemborexant.

FOR OTHER COMMON SLEEP DISORDERS

For those who suffer from central sleep apnoea, theophylline or acetazolamide may be used to stimulate breathing. Melatonin, or medications with a similar function, are used in those with insomnia and those who have an altered circadian rhythm. Supplemental iron and medicines used to treat low dopamine, such as levodopa, ropinirole and pramipexole, are used in the management of restless legs syndrome (RLS). Drugs that promote wakefulness, such as modafinil, methylphenidate and dexamphetamine, can be used to help manage narcolepsy.

COGNITIVE BEHAVIOURAL THERAPY (CBT)

CBT is a very effective tool for combating sleep difficulties. It involves challenging a person's beliefs and misconceptions about sleep and teaching sleep-promoting behaviours. It has a number of different components including:

SLEEP RESTRICTION THERAPY

Research has shown that spending too much time in bed can actually cause you to have insomnia. This is especially true for those who go to bed when they are not tired or who lie awake anxious or thinking about the day's events. Sleep restriction sets strict limits on the time you spend in bed each night. The initial limit used is the amount of time you actually spend asleep on a nightly basis and does not include the time you spend tossing and turning before you fall asleep. At first, this may cause some daytime tiredness as you will get less sleep when you start. This will increase your sleep pressure and make sleep arrive more quickly. The goal of sleep restriction therapy is to ensure that the time you spend in bed is used for sleeping and not lying awake worrying.

STIMULUS-CONTROL THERAPY

This therapy teaches you to develop positive associations between sleep and your sleep environment. Recommendations, such as getting out of bed if you can't sleep and keeping your work out of the bedroom, are used to help establish sleep-promoting connections. The goal is to only associate the bedroom with calmness, tranquility and relaxation.

PARADOXICAL INTENTION THERAPY

This therapy involves eliminating the anxiety that surrounds trying to fall asleep. Instead of attempting to sleep, a person experiencing sleeping difficulties attempts to stay awake for as long as they can. This will diminish the fear of not being able to fall asleep and help you to nod off without effort.

SLEEP EDUCATION

This helps you learn what is considered healthy and normal when it comes to sleep. Many people have unrealistic expectations about how much sleep they need and mistaken ideas about the consequences of a night or two of poor sleep. This can cause unnecessary bedtime worry, and lead to insomnia.

LIGHT THERAPY

Light therapy is used to treat those with an altered circadian rhythm and seasonal affective disorder. It involves exposing the eyes to bright natural or artificial light for a certain amount of time to help reset the circadian clock. Daylight exposure is the most natural way to regulate the internal clock, however this is not always feasible.

The most common source of light used for the therapy is a light box. The box houses light-emitting tubes and sits on top of a table. The intensity of the light is measured in lux. Most sources provide 10,000 lux of light.

During a treatment you are required to face the direction of the light box while remaining a certain distance from it for a set period of time. Treatment sessions are often about 20–30 minutes in length. The timing of the treatment depends on the condition being treated.

For DSWPD (see page 81) and seasonal affective disorder, light therapy is often administered after waking in the morning. For those who work night shifts, bright light exposure should occur in the late evening. For jet lag, the timing of light therapy depends on the direction of travel. If travelling eastwards, bright light exposure should occur in the morning after waking to advance your sleep time. If flying westwards, bright light should be administered in the evening to delay sleep onset.

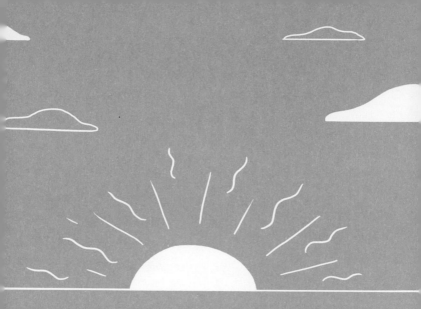

If a light box is not convenient, there are desk lamps and visors that can provide bright light. Another type of light therapy is dawn simulation. This is provided by a dawn simulator, a device that gradually increases the brightness of a room. The dawn simulator mimics a natural sunrise and helps you to wake up in a relaxed manner. Dawn simulators can be very helpful to those who have trouble waking in the morning. Dawn simulation can be used on its own or in combination with other types of light therapy for the treatment of circadian rhythm sleep-wake disorders.

BREATHING DEVICES

These are considered to be the most effective treatment for sleep apnoea. The most common is continuous positive airway pressure (CPAP). With CPAP treatment, you wear a special mask attached to a CPAP machine while you sleep. The CPAP machine blows a stream of air through the mask and into your nose and airways. The air creates pressure, which holds your airways open, so that you can breathe properly.

Recently, other devices have been developed for the treatment of sleep apnoea. Automatic positive airway pressure (APAP) can adjust the air pressure throughout the night, unlike CPAP, which delivers a continuous stream of pressurized air. Another device called bilevel positive airway pressure (BiPAP) delivers two different pressures, one for inspiration and one for expiration. Adaptive servo-ventilation (ASV) adjusts the air pressure as needed and helps to support breathing and oxygen levels.

DIETARY AND LIFESTYLE CHANGES

The foods we eat certainly have an impact on how well we sleep. A diet rich in fruits, vegetables, wholegrains, healthy fats (such as omega-3s) and good sources of protein (such as lean meats, nuts and seeds) can help to provide the many nutrients that the body needs to build hormones and support brain function. Sweets and other unhealthy foods promote alertness and lead to weight gain. Daily exercise, eliminating smoking, limiting alcohol intake and weight management can help to reduce the incidence of a number of sleep disorders.

HERBAL THERAPY

Herbal therapy can effectively bring about calmness at bedtime. Herbs that are often used to promote sleep are valerian, lemon balm, passionflower and chamomile. These can be enjoyed as a refreshing cup of tea. They are also readily available in other forms, including tablets, capsules and tincture.

Essential oils are wonderful for helping you wind down after a challenging day. Lavender, sandalwood, ylang ylang, chamomile and marjoram essential oils have calming and relaxing properties. You can add a few drops of essential oil to a warm bath, an essential oil diffuser, or a natural massage oil (such as jojoba oil or almond oil) and gently massage the back of your neck, legs or arms.

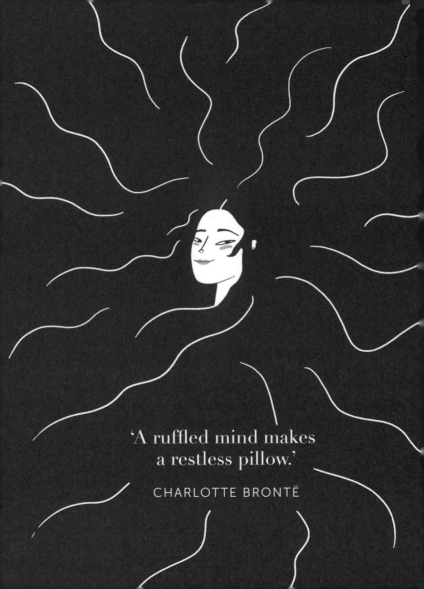

'A ruffled mind makes
a restless pillow.'

CHARLOTTE BRONTË

SHARE YOUR SLEEP STRUGGLES

Sleep problems are very common. Statistics show that many of us have experienced sleepless nights. So, why is it that we are not inclined to share the details of our bedtime tussles?

SLEEP IS UNDERVALUED

We all know that sleep is important, but most of us do not acknowledge to what degree. It is well accepted that the food we eat is essential to life, and that eating too much, not enough or unhealthy varieties can have devastating consequences. The same can be said about exercise. We all recognize that a sedentary lifestyle can predispose us to the development of a number of disorders.

The perception of sleep is quite different. In modern times, we place far less value on getting a good night's sleep than in the past. With the demands of daily life, sleep is often viewed as something that gets in the way of our to-do lists. The health consequences of chronic sleep loss take time to manifest and the symptoms of short-term sleep loss can be masked with caffeine. As a result, we tend to forget that sleep is necessary for survival.

WE FEEL THAT WE CAN MANAGE

Most of us have endured brief periods of poor sleep. We persevered through the tiredness and indulged in an extra cup or two of coffee to help us get through the day. This has given us the false impression that prolonged sleep loss can, and should, be manageable.

SLEEP LOSS IS CONSIDERED NORMAL

Technology has brought with it the end of the 8-hour work day. Many of us are often expected to respond to emails and text messages soon (usually within minutes) after we receive them. Most of us purchase goods or services online long after the shops have closed, and service providers have left for the day. We have become a 24-hour society and if the world doesn't appear to sleep, then why should we? To the detriment of our health, getting the bare minimum amount of sleep has become the new norm.

WHY TALK ABOUT SLEEP?

Talking about any problem, sleep loss included, is beneficial for a number of reasons.

IT'S GOOD FOR YOUR HEALTH

Talking about your sleep struggles can be very therapeutic. It can help to ease any sadness or worry that you are experiencing and keep the levels of stress hormones in check. Sharing any thoughts, feelings or experiences that are causing you to lose sleep can do wonders for enhancing your physical, emotional and mental health.

OTHER PEOPLE CAN RELATE

Sleep disorders are prevalent, and many are on the rise. While sharing your experiences you are likely to come across others in your life who also suffer from sleep loss. This can be very reassuring and promote healing. Those who are going through similar struggles can provide you with helpful tips as well as information on local supports and services.

IT CAN IDENTIFY OTHER HEALTH PROBLEMS

Sleep troubles can be a sign of another condition. Sharing information about your sleep difficulties in addition to other symptoms that you are experiencing can help identify other health issues. In many instances, remedying the sleep loss involves managing any other ailments that are associated with it.

THE SLEEP DIARY

Diaries provide an outlet, a place to channel our thoughts, experiences and desires. Many people are familiar with the concept of a diary, however the idea of keeping a sleep diary may seem a little peculiar. The sleep diary is a place to record everything you can about your sleep. Every morning you can write down: how long it took you to nod off; what time you fell asleep; how many times you woke during the night (and for what reason); what time you roused in the morning; and how you felt when you woke up. You should also make note of any dreams you recall, as well as how vivid and detailed they were.

A sleep diary can also include information about how you felt during the day, for example whether you were tired, or had difficulty concentrating. You can also write down any observations made by your bed partner or any suggestions or comments given to you by others.

The sleep diary is a fantastic tool to help you, your loved ones and your doctors and therapists take a deeper look at the sleep troubles you are having and determine to what degree they are affecting you and others in your life. You can write your sleep diary for as long as you wish, however most healthcare providers will often want to see 1–2 weeks' worth of sleep information.

IT'S TIME TO SHARE

FAMILY AND FRIENDS
Telling your family and friends about your sleep struggles is very important. They can be a source of reassurance and support. Being up front about your sleep problems will also provide your bed partner an opportunity to share anything they may have observed while you slept.

HEALTHCARE PROVIDERS
Talking to a doctor is vital. They are the detectives who will seek out information and use both obvious and obscure clues to help you solve your sleep mystery. They will ask questions and conduct a thorough assessment. They can also refer you for testing and supply information on the various treatment options that are available.

In addition to your doctors, it is often helpful to share your sleep struggles with other healthcare providers depending on what you are experiencing. Psychologists, psychotherapists, counsellors and naturopaths are just a few examples of practitioners who may be able to assist in remedying your sleep troubles.

YOURSELF
Being honest with yourself is key to a deep and restful night's sleep. Recognizing that you are not sleeping well and being aware that a good night's sleep is achievable, will help you to seek the guidance you need and implement the changes that will enable you to succeed.

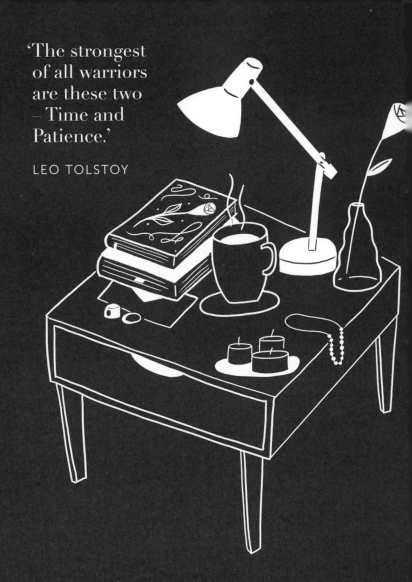

'The strongest
of all warriors
are these two
– Time and
Patience.'

LEO TOLSTOY

3 ... 2 ... 1 ... DRIFT OFF!

Sleep is a peaceful state that we inherently welcome with open arms. Sometimes, aspects of our lives get in the way of this instinctive process and we lie awake anxious and contemplative. Implementing simple changes to your daily habits and routine can allow for a smooth transition from wakefulness to sleep. Sleep hygiene is the term used to describe daytime and night-time practices and behaviours that enhance the depth and duration of sleep.

When you are ready to drift off into the realm of blissful sleep every night you should incorporate these elements:

AN ENJOYABLE AND SOOTHING RITUAL

Establishing a pleasant bedtime routine will help your body and mind wind down after a taxing day. Taking a warm bath, reading a book or listening to relaxing music each night will help condition your body to know that it's time to sleep.

A REGULAR AND GRADUAL WAKE UP

Waking up at the same time every day (including weekends and holidays) will help to create a sleep schedule. You will soon start to become tired at the same time every day. Waking up slowly will help you start the day with more energy and less sleep inertia.

A DIMINISHED DAYTIME DOZE

Sleeping during the daytime will reduce your sleep pressure and make you less tired at night. However, there are some instances where napping is helpful. Shift workers, those who suffer from narcolepsy and those who are sleep-deprived and required to drive a car or perform complex tasks, can benefit from a short (less than 30 minutes) nap.

SLEEP IS FOR THE WEARY

Lying in bed when you are not tired and ready for sleep will make you feel frustrated.

A PET-FREE BED

Avoid sleeping with your pet. An animal that makes noise or moves around during the night can negatively affect your sleep.

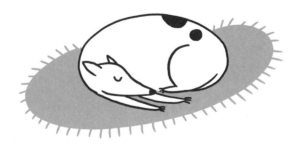

A RELAXED MIND

You should only go to bed when you are free of worry, sadness or anger. Resolve conflicts and address problems as best as you can before bedtime. Anything that is unsettled has a tendency to enter the mind while you are at rest.

EXIT THE ROOM IF SLEEP DOESN'T ARRIVE SOON

Leave your bedroom if you do not fall asleep within 20 minutes of going to bed. The best thing to do if you can't sleep is to get up, go to a dimly lit room and do a relaxing activity. Return to bed only when you are sleepy.

A BED RESERVED FOR REST

Your bed should be used for calming pursuits such as sleep and sexual activity. It is best not to watch television, use your computer, tablet or mobile phone, eat or think about the day's events in bed.

A CONCEALED CLOCK

Place your clock under, or away from, your bed. Looking at the clock during the night can be very anxiety-provoking and wreak havoc on your sleep. Put your clock in a place where you can't see it.

A SNACK-SIZED PORTION

Eating a large meal within 3 hours of going to bed can lead to digestive upset, difficulty falling asleep and frequent waking.

HUNGER WILL HINDER

You should not attempt to sleep if you are hungry. Hunger hormones will increase your alertness.

A WELL-BALANCED DIET

Nutrients such as iron, zinc, vitamin C and folic acid are required for the synthesis of melatonin. Eating a wide assortment of healthy foods will ensure that your body gets what it needs.

CAFFEINE FOR THE RISE

Only drink caffeinated beverages in the morning. The stimulating effect of caffeine can last a long time. If you find that you are highly sensitive to caffeine it may be best to avoid it altogether.

DAILY EXERCISE

Regular physical activity will build sleep pressure and enhance your overall health. You should avoid exercise within 3 hours of bedtime if you find that it makes you unable to sleep.

BE CIGARETTE-FREE

Nicotine can disrupt melatonin production.

LESS FLUID FOR ADDED SLEEP

Avoid liquids just before bed. This will reduce the likelihood of having to get up to empty your bladder during the night.

AVOID EVENING ALCOHOL

Alcohol can disrupt your sleep.

A PLAN FOR SCHEDULE ADJUSTMENTS

Prepare for travelling across time zones or a long-term (greater than one week) shift change in advance. To minimize the effects of an altered sleep schedule, gradually shift your bedtime to that of your travel destination, or to that of your new work shift wake time, more than 3–4 days in advance.

TIME TO UNWIND

Step away from your hectic schedule and take some time to notice the beauty that surrounds you.

CREATE YOUR SLEEP SANCTUARY

Your sleep environment is your place to rest and revitalize.
Here are some ways to ensure that it is conducive to a
good night's sleep.

CALMING DECORATIONS
Any photographs or artwork that you have displayed
should feature images that make you feel positive
and relaxed.

SOFT, EARTHY OR NEUTRAL WALL COLOURS
Bold colours can be very rousing and promote alertness.
Choose less vibrant colours, such as white, soft pink, light
grey, taupe, lavender, olive or baby blue.

DIM LIGHTING
Your bedroom should be free of bright lights.

COOL TEMPERATURE
To induce sleep, it is recommended that your bedroom
temperature be between 16 and 20ºC (61 and 68ºF).

COMPLETE DARKNESS
Using black-out blinds or a face mask can block out any light.

SILENCE
Loud noises can make falling asleep very difficult. If sleeping in a noisy area is unavoidable, background white noise or earplugs can help to block out sleep-disruptive sounds.

CLEAN, CLEAR AND CALM
A room that is open and uncluttered is more welcoming and relaxing. Also, when you see that your room needs tidying up, your mind immediately labels it as a task that needs to be completed. Worrying about this unfinished duty can make it more difficult to fall asleep.

FREE OF ELECTRONIC DEVICES
These emit light that can disrupt melatonin production. Many of us use our computers, tablets and mobile phones for work. These devices will therefore cause us to associate our bedroom with our work worries.

POSITION YOURSELF FOR SUCCESS

Your sleep position can have a large impact on the quality of your slumber. There are advantages and disadvantages to each of the more common sleep poses:

P: Position
A: Advantages
D: Disadvantages

PRONE (LYING ON THE STOMACH) POSITIONS

THE SECURITY POSTURE

P: Lying on your stomach with your head turned to the side and your arms wrapped around your pillow or facing forwards towards your head.

A: Eases snoring and sleep apnoea.

D: The spine is not in alignment, which can result in neck and back pain. This position can also lead to shoulder discomfort. Prone sleep positions are considered the least desirable.

THE CANDLESTICK POSTURE

P: Lying on your stomach with your head turned to the side and your arms at your sides.

A: Eases snoring and sleep apnoea.

D: Does not leave the spine in a good position and can cause neck and back pain. Prone sleep positions are considered the least desirable.

SIDE-LYING POSITIONS

THE BENCH POSTURE

P: Lying on your side with your legs straight and arms at your sides.

A: Keeps the spine straight, which can ease neck and back pain. Improves acid reflux and sleep apnoea.

D: You may involuntarily move your upper leg while you sleep, which can rotate your hip and cause pain.

THE CUDDLE POSTURE

P: Lying on your side with your legs straight and arms outwards in front of you.

A: Keeps the spine straight, which can ease neck and back pain. Improves acid reflux and sleep apnoea.

D: Puts weight on your shoulder and arm, which can lead to discomfort. Upper leg movement while you sleep can rotate the spine causing pain in your low back and hip.

THE FOETAL POSTURE

P: Lying on your side with your knees and elbows bent. This is the most common sleep position.

A: Reduces acid reflux and sleep apnoea.

D: Being curled up too tightly for a prolonged period can make your muscles sore and make breathing difficult.

SUPINE (LYING ON THE BACK) POSITIONS

THE LEADER POSTURE

P: Lying on your back with arms at your sides.

A: Puts the neck and back in comfortable positions.

D: Increases the likelihood of airway narrowing or collapse, so avoid this position if you snore or suffer from sleep apnoea. However, this position is considered the best in all other circumstances.

THE INFANT POSTURE

P: Lying on your back with your elbows bent and arms facing upwards.

A: Puts the neck and back in comfortable positions.

D: May lead to shoulder pain and worsen snoring or sleep apnoea.

THE MATTRESS MATTERS

Although personal preference is the most important factor, there are some things you should bear in mind when selecting a mattress.

- A BIGGER MATTRESS IS A BETTER MATTRESS: Purchasing a mattress that is too small is a very common mistake. Your mattress should be large enough to accommodate you (and your bed partner) and any movement or repositioning that occurs during sleep.

- A MATTRESS THAT IS TOO FIRM IS JUST AS BAD AS ONE THAT IS TOO SOFT: A mattress that is too firm can worsen pain, while one that is too soft will provide little support. A medium-firm mattress is often recommended for promoting sleep and reducing pain, however this type of mattress may not be ideal for everyone, so it is always best to test different varieties to determine which offers you the most comfort.

- THERE IS TOO MUCH HYPE AROUND THE MATTRESS TYPE: Pocket sprung, foam, latex, etc. – there are so many options. Countless adverts feature manufacturers claiming to possess a superior product. How do you know which to choose? The best way to purchase a mattress is to look at the benefits of each and determine the one that best meets your needs. Also remember that comfort is key, and the most expensive mattress is not necessarily the best mattress.

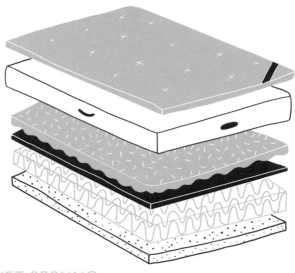

POCKET SPRUNG

This is the most popular variety. They offer comfort and support but can wear easily.

FOAM

These mattresses offer comfort and support and limit motion across the mattress. They support the natural alignment of the spine and are considered the best mattress for those who suffer from pain. Unfortunately, some foam mattresses do not breathe very well and can become quite hot. Some may also have a chemical odour.

LATEX

This variety offers comfort, support and breathability. Latex mattresses also have a long lifespan and do not retain heat. A major drawback is that they can be quite expensive.

HYBRID

This often refers to a combination of springs and foam, so they offer the benefits and drawbacks of both types. These mattresses tend to be quite expensive and many do not have a long lifespan.

ORGANIC

These are often made with organic latex, organic cotton and organic wool. They are hypoallergenic and free of potentially carcinogenic chemicals. The downside is that they tend to be expensive and may be difficult to find.

AIR

These mattresses can offer good comfort, support and pain relief. The major drawbacks are that they can lose air over time, the pump may be loud, they require assembly and they can be expensive in comparison to the other mattress types.

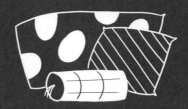

THE POWER OF THE PILLOW

Choosing the right pillow (or whether or not to use a pillow) can make the difference between a night of restful sleep and one fraught with tossing and turning. When selecting a pillow, the decision should be based on your sleep position, comfort level and personal preference.

THE STOMACH-SLEEPER
A thin pillow (or no pillow at all) is your best choice to avoid any discomfort in your neck or upper back. A second thin pillow placed under your abdomen can be used for added comfort.

THE SIDE-SLEEPER
Here, a thicker pillow is ideal. If you experience back pain, a second pillow between your knees will keep your spine in proper alignment.

THE BACK-SLEEPER
A thinner pillow is often the best choice; however, some people prefer a thick pillow to provide neck support. A pillow under your knees can help to support the spine.

FREE YOUR MIND

In order to fall asleep, your mind needs to be relaxed and free of worry. Your body must be comfortable, with your muscles relieved of all tension and your breathing slow and deep. The following simple exercises will help to put your mind and body at ease, so there is no apprehension and fear when you lie down to sleep.

CAPTURING THE MOMENT

Taking the time to examine and explore your environment will increase your awareness and your ability to focus on the here and now. You will be better able to focus on the positives and free yourself of negative emotions. You can do this exercise during the day or at night.

1. Sit in a comfortable chair, with your arms relaxed and your feet touching the ground. Select any object in your environment, such as a book or a photograph.

2. Bring your focus to that object. Notice its size, shape, colour and any other features you can observe.

3. If your mind wanders, gently bring your focus back to the object. If the object brings about strong emotions or feelings, simply acknowledge their presence and return your focus to what you are observing.

4. Remain focused on the object for 15 minutes.

GREETING THE NIGHT'S SKY

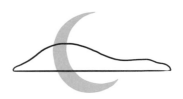

Melatonin production increases in the presence of darkness. Unfortunately, our homes and our devices immerse us in artificial light long after the sun has set. Noticing that darkness has arrived will tell your mind and body that bedtime is near and that it is time to relax.

1. Once the sun has set, enter a room with a window.

2. Turn off the light, stand at the window and gaze into the darkness.

3. Stare deeply into the night's sky.

4. Explore its emptiness and beauty.

5. Notice its calmness, peacefulness and tranquility.

6. Feel yourself being enveloped in its warm embrace.

7. Watch your worries being swept away into its infinite space.

8. When you are ready, step away from the window.

Once you have completed this exercise it is best to keep the lights in your environment dim and avoid using devices that emit artificial light until the morning.

STRETCHING FOR SLEEP

Stretching your muscles before you sleep can relax your mind, ease tension, enhance circulation and support spinal alignment.

THE FLOWER BLOSSOM

Lie on your back and bring yourself into the foetal position, with your arms tightly grasping your legs and your chin tucked in. Take a deep breath in, hold for 10 seconds, and as you exhale gently release your arms and legs. Take another deep breath in, hold for 10 seconds and as you exhale, slowly bring your arms up over your head, extend your legs with your toes pointed and curve your back as it rises. Hold for 10 seconds.

THE BOW STRETCH

Sit with your back straight, your legs out in front of you and your arms at your sides. Gently bring your arms up until your fingers are reaching for the sky. Then slowly bend forward with your arms stretched. Tuck your chin into your chest. Hold for 15 seconds.

THE SPINE TWIST

Lie on your back with your arms behind your head. Place your feet flat on the floor with your knees bent. While keeping your knees and feet together, and without moving your upper back, lower your knees to one side. Hold for 20 seconds. Lower your knees to the other side and hold for 20 seconds.

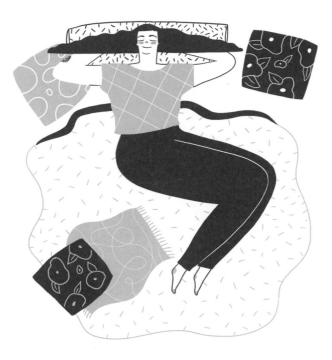

THE SLEEPER'S BREATH

Slow, regular and rhythmic breathing is important for the early sleep stages. The Sleeper's Breath is a controlled breathing exercise that helps to calm the mind and prepare the body to enter stage 1 sleep. Make sure you inhale and exhale through your nose while taking your deep breaths. Nose breathing enhances oxygen levels and can reduce the occurrence of snoring and sleep apnoea.

1. Lie down on your bed.

2. Close your eyes.

3. Place your right hand on your upper chest and your left hand on your abdomen.

4. Take a deep breath in, hold for a count of four, then slowly exhale. Do three more of these breaths.

5. Take a deep breath in hold for a count of six, then slowly exhale. Do three more of these breaths.

6. Take a deep breath in, hold for a count of eight, then slowly exhale. Continue these breaths until you feel relaxed and ready to drift off.

BEDTIME MEDITATION

Meditation for sleep has two purposes: to calm your mind, and to turn your sleep environment into a place of relaxation and tranquility.

1. Lie down on your bed.

2. Take a deep breath in through your nose, hold for 4 seconds, then slowly exhale through your nose. Do three more of these breaths.

3. Notice the bed beneath you, feel yourself sinking into its warmth and allow it to envelop and protect you.

4. Look at the walls that surround you. These are your defenders, shielding your sanctuary and providing you with comfort and tranquility.

5. Nothing can enter your shelter, nothing will disturb your peace, you are free.

6. Feel the calmness and serenity of your room, you are safe, you are secure.

RELEASING MUSCLE TENSION

Easing muscle tension involves tensing and relaxing each muscle group. This type of exercise, known as a progressive muscle relaxation, will relieve stress and help your body enter sleep. Make sure you inhale and exhale through your nose while taking your deep breaths.

1. Sit on a soft, comfortable chair or lie down on your bed.

2. Close your eyes and place your right hand on your abdomen.

3. Take a deep breath in, hold for 10 seconds, then slowly exhale. Do three more of these breaths. Place your right hand at your side.

4. Bring your attention to your toes and your feet. Take a deep breath in and, while you do, tense the muscles in your feet and toes. Curl your toes and feel the tension deep in the soles of your feet. Hold the breath for 10 seconds, then slowly relax the muscles as you exhale.

5. Bring your attention to the muscles in your lower legs. Take a deep breath in and tense all of the muscle groups in your lower legs. Hold the breath for 10 seconds and feel the tightness in your calf muscles. Slowly relax the muscles as you exhale.

6. Bring your attention to the muscles in your thighs and buttocks. Take a deep breath in and tense all of these

muscles. Hold the breath for 10 seconds. Slowly exhale and feel the warmth as you allow the muscles to relax.

7. Bring your attention to your stomach. Take a deep breath in and tighten your stomach muscles. Hold the breath for 10 seconds. Then, slowly exhale and let the tension go.

8. Bring your attention to your back. Take a deep breath in and tense all of the muscles in your upper and lower back. Tilt your head back slightly as you are tensing these muscles. Hold the breath for 10 seconds, then slowly relax the muscles and bring your head forward as you exhale.

9. Bring your attention to your arms. Take a deep breath in and tense your arm muscles. Make a tight fist and bend your arms at your elbows. Hold the breath for 10 seconds, then slowly relax the muscles as you exhale. Unclench your fists and place your arms at your side.

10. Bring your attention to your shoulders. Take a deep breath in and tense your shoulder muscles by bringing them up as if you are shrugging your shoulders. Hold the breath for 10 seconds, then slowly relax the muscles as you exhale.

11. Bring your attention to your neck muscles. Take a deep breath in and tighten these muscles while tilting your head back. Hold the breath for 10 seconds, then slowly relax the muscles and bring your head forward as you exhale.

12. Bring your attention to your forehead. Take a deep breath and open your eyes as wide as you can. Hold the breath for 10 seconds, then slowly exhale, close your eyes and relax.

13. Bring your attention to your jaw. Take a deep breath and open your mouth as wide as you can. Hold the breath for 10 seconds, then slowly exhale, close your mouth and relax.

14. Place your right hand on your abdomen and take a deep breath in, hold for 10 seconds, then slowly exhale. Do three more of these breaths.

15. Open your eyes.

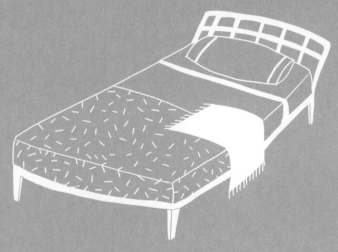

FREEING THE SPIRIT

In traditional Chinese medicine, the heart is the organ that houses the spirit. Disharmony and imbalances in the organ manifest as nervousness, sadness and poor sleep. The heart meridian runs along the inner arm originating just below the shoulder and terminating at the edge of your little finger. This exercise is a gentle self-massage to bring the heart back into balance.

1. Sit in a comfortable chair, with your elbows bent and your arms resting on your thighs with palms facing upwards.

2. Take the index and middle fingers of your right hand and lightly massage the inner aspect of your upper left arm in a circular motion. Continue this soothing motion down the length of your arm to the top of your hand and down to your little finger. Repeat this motion three times.

3. Use your entire right palm to slowly stroke the full length of your inner left arm and hand, from your shoulder to your fingertips. Repeat this motion three times.

4. Repeat the exercise on the right arm.

TENSION RELEASE (CLENCHED FISTS)

This is a very quick and effective exercise that you can do to alleviate stress and worry.

1. Sit in a comfortable chair and place your hands in front of you, with your elbows bent and thumbs pointed upwards.

2. Close your eyes and visualize all of your anxieties and worries travelling down from your neck and shoulders into your hands.

3. Take a deep breath in and clench your fists. Hold for 15 seconds.

4. As you exhale, unclench your fists while turning your palms face up. Feel the negative energy escaping from your body.

5. Take another deep breath, hold for 15 seconds, and then slowly exhale.

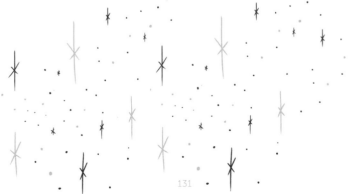

THE MORNING RISE

Many of us wake up to the sound of an alarm and are forced to quickly leap out of bed and begin the day. Rousing in the morning should be gradual with time to breathe and awaken your senses. Stretching first thing is a great way to ease muscle stiffness and increase blood circulation. This exercise is a simple morning stretch routine that will help to increase your alertness and release any tension that emerged while you slept.

1. When you wake from sleep, take a deep breath in, hold for 10 seconds, then slowly exhale. Focus on the sound of your breathing. Do three more of these breaths.

2. With your knees straight and back remaining on the bed, gently raise your legs as high as you comfortably can. Hold for 10 seconds, then release.

3. Sit up and raise your arms above your head. Reach up as high as you can and hold for 10 seconds.

4. While remaining seated, bend at your waist to the left, return to the centre, turn to the right and then back to the centre. Lower your arms.

5. Bring your chin to your chest, hold for 10 seconds, then bring your head back to the centre. Repeat while gently tilting your head back, turning your head to the left, turning your head to the right, bringing your left

ear to your left shoulder and bringing your right ear to your right shoulder.

6. Extend and gently stretch both of your legs, hold for 10 seconds.

7. Reach your left arm over to your right leg to touch the toes of your right foot. Hold for 10 seconds. Repeat with the right arm and left leg, then release.

8. Take a deep breath in, hold for 10 seconds, then slowly exhale. Do three more of these breaths.

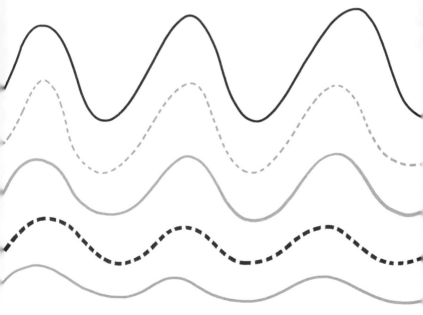

STRESS LESS, SLEEP MORE

Sometimes the stresses of everyday life can be overwhelming. Feeling trapped in a difficult situation or overcome by negative emotions can have a profound effect on our bodies and our minds.

When stress takes hold, we feel confined. We cannot think clearly or reason. Our hearts race as we seek to escape.

When we are weakened by distress, we must close our eyes, tune in to our senses and remember to breathe.

MANAGING BEDTIME WORRY

The nervousness that we bring with us to bed will make falling asleep and staying asleep very challenging. Exploring our worries and engaging in self-reflection can help to dissipate our night-time tensions.

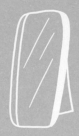

REFLECTIVE QUESTIONS

- What happens to my body when I am overpowered by negative thoughts?

- What unhelpful situations do I need to avoid?

- What will comfort me during times of stress?

- How can I take time away from those things that upset me?

- Where or to whom can I turn when I feel overwhelmed?

THE PROBLEM-SOLVING AND PLANNING WORKSHEET

This is a simple exercise that will help you navigate through any struggles that you have. The Problem-Solving and Planning Worksheet provides a place and an opportunity to contemplate, plan, record and heal.

At least 3 hours before bedtime, find a place that is quiet and calm.

1. Take a piece of paper and draw a line down the centre.

2. On the left-hand side list all of your worrying thoughts and unsolved problems.

3. Take some time to think about why those anxiety-provoking thoughts came about and what actions you can take to mitigate them. You can also ponder ways (or next steps) to resolve the problems that you have listed on this side of the page.

4. Write these actions on the right-hand side of the page beside the corresponding worrying thought or problem.

Not only does this activity encourage you to think through all of your troublesome thoughts, but should you find yourself awake at night pondering, referring back to the Problem-Solving and Planning Worksheet is a great way to remind yourself that you have thought about, and decided upon, steps to be taken to solve the worries or problems that are keeping you from sleeping.

CONQUERING YOUR SLEEP ANXIETIES

Any thoughts or beliefs that you have about sleep can influence the amount of sleep you will get. If you tell yourself that you must get 8 hours of sleep in order to function and any less would be devastating to your daytime performance, it is quite likely that you will continue to lie awake well into the night. This situation is often brought on by misconceptions and misinformation about how much sleep we truly need.

Similarly, when you go to bed anxious and fearful about not being able to fall asleep, the result will tend to be a night of poor sleep. This anticipatory anxiety about not sleeping, and the consequences of not sleeping, is very common.

In reality, humans are very resilient beings and brief disruptions in the sleep-wake cycle do not usually lead to serious health consequences. At times, life can get in the way of a good night's sleep. If you lose a night of sleep, your body will do what it can to get the rest that it needs. Your body will use important cues, such as making you feel tired earlier than usual the following night, to tell you when it's an ideal time to go to bed.

Sleep is a beautiful time that allows us to rest and revive. Embrace this magical state and enjoy it to its fullest. I bid you sound sleep and blissful dreams.

SAFETY NOTES

This material is presented for information and for educational purposes only. If you suffer from recurring sleeping difficulties or night-time awakenings you should seek medical attention. If you or your bed partner notice any unusual occurrences while you are falling asleep, during sleep or upon rousing, you should also obtain medical advice. Poor sleep can be a symptom of an underlying condition, so it is always advisable to have your disrupted sleep investigated.

The medications, bright lights, herbal preparations, sleep restriction, exercises and other therapies described in this book can have undesirable side-effects and negative interactions and are not recommended for use by those who suffer from certain health conditions or who have undergone recent surgeries. All of the treatments discussed in this book should only be used under the guidance and supervision of a physician.

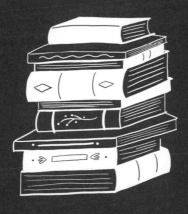

QUOTES WERE TAKEN FROM

E. Joseph Cossman was an American entrepreneur. He marketed a number of successful products and authored books on how to succeed in business.

Moira Young is a Canadian novelist best known as the author of *Blood Red Road*, *Rebel Heart* and *Raging Star*.

William Shakespeare was an English poet and playwright. His many works, including *Macbeth*, *Richard III*, *Romeo and Juliet* and *Hamlet,* continue to be celebrated and enjoyed by readers and audiences throughout the world.

William Penn was an English philosopher and entrepreneur. He founded the Province of Pennsylvania in English North America.

Thomas Dekker was an English playwright. He wrote and cowrote a number of plays including *The Pleasant Comedie of Old Fortunatus*, *The Shoemaker's Holiday or the Gentle Craft*, *The Virgin Martyr* and *The Witch of Edmonton*.

Clifton Fadiman was an American author and radio and television personality. His books include *Fantasia Mathematica*, *The Mathematical Magpie* and *The Lifetime Reading Plan*.

Charlotte Brontë was an English poet and novelist. Her works include *Jane Eyre*, *Shirley* and *Villette*.

Leo Tolstoy was a Russian writer, philosopher and political thinker. His works include *War and Peace, The Cossacks* and *Anna Karenina*.

SELECTED BIBLIOGRAPHY

Billiard, Michel and Chokroverty, Sudhansu. *Sleep Medicine: A Comprehensive Guide to Its Development, Clinical Milestones, and Advances in Treatment*. New York. Springer-Verlag. 2015.

Clarysse, Willy, Schoors, Antoon and Quaegebeur, Jan. *Egyptian Religion: The Last Thousand Years*. Leuven. Peeters Publishers. 1998.

Crick, Francis and Mitchison, Graeme. 'The function of dream sleep'. *Nature*. 1983. 304, 111–114

Ekirch, A. Roger. *At Day's Close: Night in Times Past*. New York. W.W. Norton & Company. 2006.

Hobson, John A. and McCarley, Robert W. 'The brain as a dream state generator: an activation-synthesis hypothesis of the dream process'. *American Journal of Psychiatry*. 1977. 134, 1335–1348

The International Classification of Sleep Disorders – Third Edition (ICSD-3). American Academy of Sleep Medicine. Darien, Illinois. 2014.

Lange, Tanja, Dimitrov, Stoyan and Born, Jan. 'Effects of sleep and circadian rhythm on the human immune system'. Annals of the New York Academy of Sciences. 2010. 1193: 48–59.

McNamara, Patrick, McLaren, Deirdre, Smith, Dana, Brown, Ariel and Stickgold, Robert. 'A "Jekyll and Hyde" within: aggressive versus friendly interactions in REM and non-REM dreams'. *Psychological Science*. 2005. 16(2), 130–136.

Nissin, Laura. *Roman Sleep: Sleeping areas and sleeping arrangements in the Roman House*. University of Helsinki. 2016.

Revonsuo, Antti. 'The reinterpretation of dreams: an evolutionary hypothesis of the function of dreaming'. *Behavioral Brain Science*. 2000. 23 (6).

Siegel, Jerome M. 'The neurotransmitters of sleep'. *The Journal of Clinical Psychiatry*. 2004. 65 Suppl. 16. 4–7.

Zhang, Jie. 'Continual-activation theory of dreaming'. *Dynamical Psychology*. 2005.

ABOUT THE AUTHOR

My journey into the world of sleep began over 20 years ago. As a youth I struggled with unrelenting delayed sleep-wake phase disorder and insomnia. Through much research and determination, I was able to overcome my sleeping difficulties using natural therapies. This led me on a mission to support others who struggle to achieve deep and restful sleep. As a Naturopath, I design and implement sleep programmes to enable individuals to regain their sleep and enjoy their lives to the fullest.

ACKNOWLEDGEMENTS

I would like to thank all of my mentors at the Canadian College of Naturopathic Medicine and the University of Toronto. I would especially like to thank Rabia Karim Meghji, Diane Peters and Mandy Seifi for their support. To my parents, who were my inspiration and whose encouragement and kindness led me on my path of healing. To my husband Ken and my little Jonah and Sierra for being patient, loving and a source of wonderful dreams.

Publishing Director Sarah Lavelle
Editor Harriet Butt
Designer Emily Lapworth
Illustrator Elda Broglio
Production Controller Sinead Hering
Production Director Vincent Smith

Published in 2019 by Quadrille,
an imprint of Hardie Grant Publishing.

Quadrille
52–54 Southwark Street
London SE1 1UN
quadrille.com

Cataloguing in Publication Data: a catalogue record
for this book is available from the British Library.

Reprinted in 2019 (twice)
10 9 8 7 6 5 4 3

ISBN: 978 1 78713 276 4

Printed in China